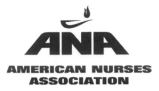

AMERICAN NURSES
ASSOCIATION

W9-BQK-600

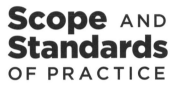

Scope AND
Standards
OF PRACTICE

Public Health
Nursing

2ND EDITION

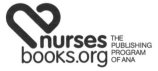

nurses THE
PUBLISHING
books.org PROGRAM
OF ANA

American Nurses Association
Silver Spring, Maryland
2013

American Nurses Association
8515 Georgia Avenue, Suite 400
Silver Spring, MD 20910-3492
1-800-274-4ANA
http://www.NursingWorld.org

Published by Nursesbooks.org
The Publishing Program of ANA
http://www.Nursesbooks.org/

The American Nurses Association (ANA) is a national professional association. This ANA publication—*Public Health Nursing: Scope and Standards of Practice, Second Edition*—reflects the thinking of the practice specialty of public health nursing on various issues and should be reviewed in conjunction with state board of nursing policies and practices. State law, rules, and regulations govern the practice of nursing, while *Public Health Nursing: Scope and Standards of Practice, Second Edition*, guides public health registered nurses in the application of their professional skills and responsibilities.

The American Nurses Association (ANA) is the only full-service professional organization representing the interests of the nation's 3.1 million registered nurses through its constituent/state nurses associations and its organizational affiliates. The ANA advances the nursing profession by fostering high standards of nursing practice, promoting the rights of nurses in the workplace, projecting a positive and realistic view of nursing, and by lobbying the Congress and regulatory agencies on healthcare issues affecting nurses and the public.

ISBN-13: 978-1-55810-490-7   SAN: 851-3481   1,000   02/14R

First printing: August 2013
Second printing: October 2013
Third printing: February 2014

Contents

Contributors

Public Health Nursing Scope and Standards Workgroup

Pamela A. Kulbok, DNSc, RN, PHCNS-BC, FAAN, Co-Chair

Joy Reed, EdD, RN, FAAN, Co-Chair

Veronica Barcelona de Mendoza, MSN, MPH, RN, APHN-BC

Sharon B. Canclini, RN, MS, FCN, CNE

Marion Donohoe, DNP, APRN, CPNP-PC

Joyce K. Edmonds, RN, MPH, PhD

Ruth N. Knollmueller, PhD, RN

Joan E. Kub, PhD, MA, PHCNS, BC

Pamela F. Levin, PhD, APHN-BC

Jeanne A. Matthews, PhD, RN

R. Adm. Kerry Paige Nesseler, MS, RN

Kathlynn Northrup-Snyder, PhD, CNS, RN

Shirley Orr, MHS, ARNP, CNAA

Capt. Sylvia Trent-Adams, PhD, MS, RN

ANA Staff

Carol Bickford, PhD, RN-BC, CPHIMS – Content editor

Maureen Cones, Esq. – Legal counsel

Katherine C. Brewer, MSN, RN – Content editor

Yvonne Humes, MSA – Project coordinator

Eric Wurzbacher, BA – Project editor

About the American Nurses Association

The American Nurses Association (ANA) is the only full-service professional organization representing the interests of the nation's 3.1 million registered nurses through its constituent/state nurses associations and its organizational affiliates. The ANA advances the nursing profession by fostering high standards of nursing practice, promoting the rights of nurses in the workplace, projecting a positive and realistic view of nursing, and by lobbying the Congress and regulatory agencies on healthcare issues affecting nurses and the public.

About Nursesbooks.org, the Publishing Program of ANA

Nursesbooks.org publishes books on ANA core issues and programs, including ethics, leadership, quality, specialty practice, advanced practice, and the profession's enduring legacy. Best known for the foundational documents of the profession on nursing ethics, scope and standards of practice, and social policy, Nursesbooks.org is the publisher for the professional, career-oriented nurse, reaching and serving nurse educators, administrators, managers, and researchers as well as staff nurses in the course of their professional development.

Scope of Public Health Nursing Practice

Public Health Nursing: Past, Present, and Future

For more than a century, public health nursing (PHN) has significantly contributed to the population's health by creating effective partnerships. Beginning in the early part of the 20th century, Lillian Wald, Lavinia Dock, and their nursing colleagues at the Henry Street Settlement House in New York's Lower East Side employed spirited innovation to organize themselves and others, working in and with communities to heal, partner, mobilize, support, and bring about change among the disadvantaged populations in which they lived and worked. Partnerships continue today as public health nurses work with communities and populations to identify specific public health assets and needs. Public health nurses address assets and needs at multiple levels, and use the political process to assure the health of communities and populations.

The health of the population is the cornerstone of public health nursing practice, as clearly described since the first iteration of this document in 1986. However, over the past few years, the terms *population health* and *population foci* have been used in other healthcare and education venues. In some cases, the use of the term *population* is intended to describe narrower specialty patient groups that the professional serves. The most notable example in nursing is the Consensus Model for APRN Regulation (APRN Joint Dialogue Group, 2008). The Consensus Model uses the term "population foci" to describe the specific patient demographics or health conditions that are the central elements of an advanced practice registered nurse's education, licensure, and certification. *Public Health Nursing; Scope and Standards of Practice, Second Edition*, describes how the focus on population health is conceptualized and actualized in the public health nursing specialty.

Public health nursing practice in the United States is dynamic and increasingly complex. Societal and political changes leading into the 21st century have enhanced this evolution. Identified threats to the health of populations include:

- Re-emergence of communicable diseases and increasing incidences of drug-resistant organisms

- Environmental hazards

- Physical or civic barriers to healthy lifestyles (e.g., food "deserts")

- Overall concern about the structure and function of the healthcare system

- Challenges imposed by the presence of modern public health epidemics such as pandemic influenza, obesity, and tobacco-related diseases and deaths

- Global and emerging crises with increased opportunities for exposure to multiple health threats

These threats have created a dramatic shift in the focus of health care toward public health all-hazards preparedness, with the ultimate goal of enhancing response and recovery. Public health nurses acquire skills in activities centered around preparedness, such as community-wide syndromic surveillance; triage and coordination of disaster health services and shelters; and the handling of biological and chemical agents as evidentiary material, as well as for the removal of a public health hazard. Innovative partnerships with community-level organizations and groups, such as communication experts, postal workers, law enforcement personnel, and other "first responders" are necessary to protect people and communities.

As priority public health initiatives evolve to address emerging health trends, public health nurses take leadership roles. They identify evidence by which new public health systems changes are implemented and evaluated, and develop operational systems that may be effectively deployed. Public health nursing leadership ultimately enhances the ability of public health systems to address the health issues facing all people and creates conditions in which people can be healthy.

Definition of Public Health Nursing

Public health nursing practice focuses on population health through continuous surveillance and assessment of the multiple determinants of health with the intent to promote health and wellness; prevent disease, disability, and premature death; and improve neighborhood quality of life. These population health priorities are addressed through identification, implementation, and evaluation of universal and targeted evidence-based programs and services that provide primary, secondary, and tertiary preventive interventions. Public health nursing practice emphasizes primary prevention with the goal of achieving health equity.

Public Health Nursing Practice: Focus on Population Health

Public health nursing practice is evidence-based and focuses on promotion of the health of entire populations and prevention of disease, injury, and premature death. Public health nursing interventions are not limited to those who seek services, are poor, or are otherwise vulnerable. Public health nurses practice in diverse settings through public, private, and nongovernmental organizations that serve populations of interest. These target populations may be at risk for, or experience, a disproportionate burden of poor health outcomes. Public health nurses partner with communities to promote, maintain, and restore health and to reduce health risks when needed healthcare services are not available. Public health nurses advocate for systems-level changes to improve health. Public health nursing services and programs may be directed toward individuals and families, groups, communities, or systems. When addressing the health of individuals and families, PHN practice is in the context of the whole population's health.

In public health nursing, *population* refers to the total number of people living in a specific geographic area (e.g., town, city, state, region, nation, multinational region). A *community* is a set of people in interaction, who may or may not share a sense of place or belonging, and who act intentionally for a common purpose (e.g., live in a neighborhood; work at a given company; or share a common cultural or demographic characteristic, health condition, or threat to health); examples include the Latino community, refugees from Somalia, women who have experienced gender discrimination, persons with mental illness, victims of a disaster. *Subpopulations, groups,* or *aggregates* consist of people experiencing a specific health condition (e.g., diseases, disabilities, pregnancy); engaging in behaviors that have the potential to negatively affect health (e.g., smoking tobacco); or sharing a common risk factor or risk exposure, or experiencing an emerging health threat or risk (e.g., victims of a disaster or a disease outbreak).

Public health nurses partner with others to achieve improved overall health of the population. Work to achieve this goal is focused using the ecological model and grounded in an awareness of multiple determinants of health, health equity, and social justice issues. This work is further supported with health behavior theories that focus on the individual, the interpersonal, community building and organizing, health communications, diffusion of ideas, and evaluation strategies.

The work of public health nurses with individuals and families is informed by the broader context of the community and/or the population. Improvement of population health is accomplished through individual health promotion strategies to increase knowledge; explore health attitudes, beliefs, and values; and facilitate behavior change to optimize personal health. Similarly, health promotion activities with families and communities are directed at shifting norms by exploring attitudes, increasing awareness, and creating group behavioral changes toward healthier alternatives in collaboration with the group. Population-level care targets laws, regulations, organizations, systems, and policies by working with key stakeholders to influence health and social conditions and ultimately optimize the population's health.

The Art and Science of Public Health Nursing: A Synergy

The unique and distinguishing characteristic of public health nursing practice, consistent with that of all public health professionals, is the focus on population health (IOM, 2003a). Another distinguishing characteristic of public health nursing practice is the goal of improving population health with the emphasis on health promotion, disease prevention, and risk reduction. Thus, the setting is not the defining characteristic of public health nursing, regardless of the terminology used to describe the public health nurse (the term *community health nurse* might still be used). Although not all public health nurses work in community settings, partnering with populations is the cornerstone of public health nursing practice.

Much as all nursing is "a learned professional built on a core body of knowledge that reflects its dual components of science and art" (ANA, 2010), public health nursing is built on a core of several systems of practice that is integrated into a whole greater than the sum of its parts. This section describes and diagrams each of these systems, and presents their resulting synergy in Figure 6 (see pg. 12).

PUBLIC HEALTH NURSING STANDARDS AND CORE COMPETENCIES

The ANA Standards of Public Health Nursing Practice are delineated in this document on pages 28–64. The competencies that accompany these 17 standards have been written largely to ensure that public health nursing fits within the domain of an ANA-recognized nursing specialty. They are diagrammed in Figure 1 below.

FIGURE 1. ANA Standards of Public Health Nursing Practice

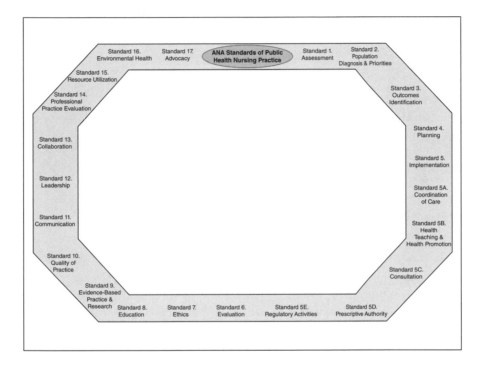

The Core Competencies for Public Health Nursing (Quad Council, 2011), organized by eight PHN practice domains, which are discussed later in the section Tiers (Levels) of Public Health Nursing Practice on pages ab–bc and in Appendix A, which starts on pg. 73. They are diagrammed in Figure 2 on the next page 6.

FIGURE 2. Core Competencies for Public Health Nursing

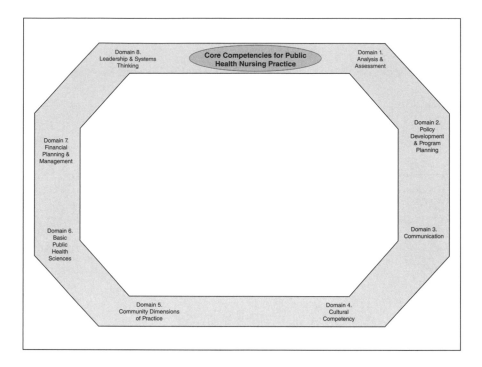

ESSENTIAL PUBLIC HEALTH SERVICES

In 1994, a CDC steering committee comprised of representatives from U.S. Public Health Service agencies and other major public health organizations, developed a set ten essential services to provide a working definition of the core function of public health and a guiding framework for the responsibilities of community public health systems (CDC, 2010). These services follow:

1. Monitor health status to identify and solve community health problems.

2. Diagnose and investigate health problems and health hazards in the community.

3. Inform, educate, and empower people about health issues.

4. Mobilize community partnerships and action to identify and solve health problems.

5. Develop policies and plans that support individual and community health efforts.

6. Enforce laws and regulations that protect health and ensure safety.

7. Link people to needed personal health services and assure the provision of health care when otherwise unavailable.

8. Assure competent public and personal healthcare workforce.

9. Evaluate effectiveness, accessibility, and quality of personal and population-based health services.

10. Research for new insights and innovative solutions to health problems.

These services are diagrammed in Figure 3

FIGURE 3. Essential Public Health Services

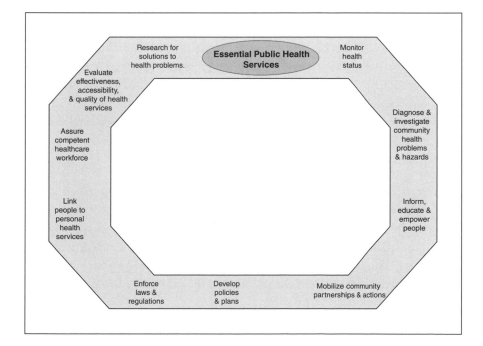

PRINCIPLES OF PUBLIC HEALTH NURSING PRACTICE

Public health nursing practice is guided by adherence to **all** of the following eight principles (Quad Council, 1997):

- *The client or unit of care is the population.* Although a public health nurse may engage in activities with individuals, families, or groups, the dominant responsibility is to the population as a whole.

- *The primary obligation is to achieve the greatest good for the greatest number of people or the population as a whole.* Public health nurses recognize that it may not be possible to meet individual needs if those needs conflict with priority health goals that benefit the whole population.

- *Public health nurses collaborate with the client as an equal partner.* The public health nurse's actions must reflect awareness of the need for comprehensive health planning in partnership with communities and populations. This includes understanding the perspectives, priorities, and values of the population when interpreting the data, making policy and program decisions, and selecting appropriate strategies for action.

- *Primary prevention is the priority in selecting appropriate activities.* Primary prevention includes health promotion and health protection strategies.

- *Public health nursing focuses on strategies that create healthy environmental, social, and economic conditions in which populations may thrive.* Public health nursing interventions include education, community development, social engineering, policy development, and enforcement. Such interventions emerge from collaboration with the population and result in laws and rules, policies, and budget priorities. An essential strategy is advocating for and teaching advocacy skills to others to create healthy conditions.

- *A public health nurse is obligated to actively identify and reach out to all who might benefit from a specific activity or service.* Because risk factors are not randomly distributed, specific subpopulations may be more vulnerable to disease or disability or may have more difficulty in accessing or using services. This requires special outreach beyond those who may present for services, to include the entire population.

- *Optimal use of available resources and creation of new evidence-based strategies is necessary to assure the best overall improvement in the health of the population.* The key components include: organizing and coordinating action responses to health issues; utilizing and providing evidence-based and cost-effectiveness information to decision-makers related to outcomes of specific actions, programs, or policies; and researching and designing the collection of evidence to ground the practice of population-based care.

■ *Collaboration with other professions, populations, organizations, and stakeholder groups is the most effective way to promote and protect the health of the people.* Creating the conditions for optimizing health is an extremely complex, resource-intensive process. To do this, public health nurses join with experts from a variety of fields and professions—and community members are seen as local experts. Leadership in this effort recognizes the importance of legislative action and involvement in the healthcare system or government health and social policy agendas at all levels.

These principles are diagrammed below in Figure 4.

FIGURE 4. Principles of Public Health Nursing Practice

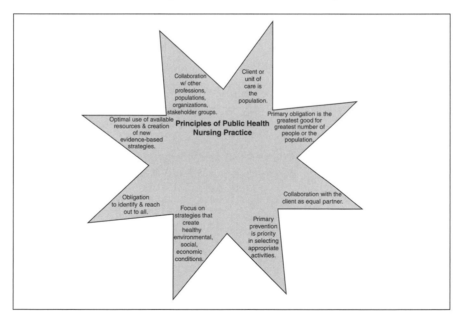

CORE FUNCTIONS OF PUBLIC HEALTH NURSING

Public health nursing practice involves application of the *core functions of public health*—assessment, assurance, and policy development—originally defined to clarify the government's role in fulfilling the mission of public health (IOM, 1988). Public health nurses adhere to these functions and the standards for public health nursing. Each function is used in a systematic and comprehensive manner to achieve optimal health goals and is carried out in partnership with the public and other key stakeholders. As leaders and advocates in these functions, public health nurses are proactive on healthcare and social issues, build effective strategies, and effect change.

- *Assessment* includes review of the concerns, strengths, and expectations of the population and is guided by epidemiological methods and the nursing process. Assessment uses both qualitative data and quantitative data.

- *Assurance* is accomplished through regulation, advocating for interdisciplinary services, coordination of community services, and (at times) direct provision of services. Assurance strategies take into account the availability, acceptability, accessibility, effectiveness, and quality of services.

- *Policy development* is accomplished through the results of assessment, identification of the population's priorities, and consideration of other subpopulations and communities at greatest risk, using effective and evidence-based strategies.

These core elements are diagrammed below in Figure 5.

FIGURE 5. Core Functions of Public Health Nursing

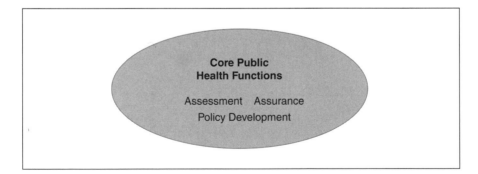

The Core Public Health Functions Steering Committee further developed the ten essential services in 1994 to provide a working definition of the core function of public health and a guiding framework for the responsibilities of community public health systems (CDC, 2010).

A SYNERGY OF SYSTEMS

Public health nurses promote the health of the public through the art and science of public health nursing practice, which is effectively the synergy of the inter-relationships and interactions of constituent systems of practice noted above as illustrated in Figure 6. This diagram is constructed to emphasize that the public health functions are at the core of PHN practice and the eight principles, which emerge from those core functions, permeate and inform all of public health nursing practice. In summary, from the center outward, these systems are:

- The three core functions of public health

- The eight principles of public health nursing practice

- The ten essential public health services.

- The Core Competencies of Public Health Nursing Practice, organized by eight practice domains

- The ANA Standards of Professional Public Health Nursing and their accompanying competencies

Thus, Figure 6 (see next page), which depicts the art and science of public health nursing practice, provides a useful framework that integrates multiple systems—standards, competencies, essential services, principles, and core functions—that are directed toward the goal of improving population health.

FIGURE 6. The Art and Science of Public Health Nursing Practice: A Synergy of Systems

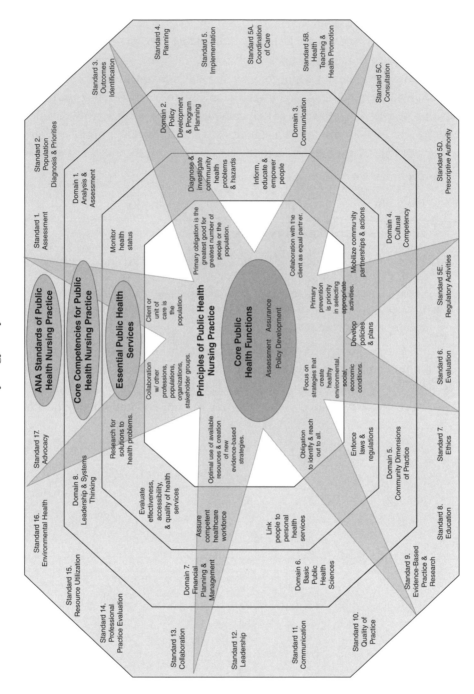

Public Health Nursing Practice: Application and Context

EVIDENCE-BASED PRACTICE

Public health nursing integrates the best current evidence with professional expertise and community or stakeholder preferences and values for improvement in population health status. Public health nurses engage in research that enhances the science and evidence base for practice and documents the outcomes of specific activities and strategies.

To be most effective and tailor the population assessments, strategies, and evaluations to the unique needs of a given population, it is important for the public health nurse to utilize a broad variety of sources of evidence. In addition to published research and evidence for utilization, the public health nurse gathers qualitative information from interviews with the community or population, documents observations of the population and the geographic locale, and explores local information such as media. Integrating this observational and ethnographic evidence with published research and other sources of data helps the public health nurse develop the breadth and depth of knowledge specific to the population being served. This base of clear and well-documented evidence permits use of the most efficient, effective, and cost-beneficial strategies to promote the public's health. Micro and macro approaches to work with populations allow the public health nurse to incorporate new questions and observations into current and previous research, thereby creating deeper understanding of the issues and identifying new areas for research.

The significant allocation of federal dollars to stimulate the infusion of health information technology into practice has generated new data and information resources, electronic and personal health records (EHRs and PHRs), enhanced connectivity via health information exchanges, electronic immunization and other registries, and other electronic capabilities. Innovative research and surveillance activities using geographic information systems (GISs) are evolving into requisite practices, for example, in community assessment and emergency preparedness initiatives.

Implementation of research and publication are essential for continuing growth in the field of public health nursing and benefit from enhanced funding resources that support studies focused on population health. Public health nurses have a responsibility to actively contribute to the bodies of knowledge of nursing, public health nursing, and public health, including the dissemination of findings.

PRACTICE ENVIRONMENTS

The focus of public health nursing practice is on population health; therefore, it often occurs in communities and other nontraditional healthcare settings. Traditionally, public health nurses were associated with governmental agencies, such as state, local, and tribal health departments. However, this specialty is now found in many venues, including some acute and primary care settings with targeted population health agendas. Public health nurses work in a variety of settings, including but not limited to: community-based or faith-based organizations, community health centers, correctional facilities, educational systems, elder care agencies, global/international agencies or organizations, health departments, health maintenance organizations, individual homes, the military, public or private clinics, schools, wellness and other outreach centers within health systems, and worksites.

In both urban and rural areas, public health nurses plan and carry out population-based interventions that are unique to community- and population-based settings. Particularly in small rural communities, public health nursing practice is often largely independent, relying on the nurse's knowledge in the field and often without the immediate support of the healthcare team.

CHARACTERISTICS OF RECIPIENTS OF PUBLIC HEALTH NURSING SERVICES

Public health nurses care for populations, which include individuals, families, groups, and communities. Even when an intervention is carried out with an individual, public health nurses have the larger population aggregate or "big picture" in mind. Individual care in public health nursing settings includes interventions such as case management and home visiting for high-risk populations. Care coordination and referral of high-risk clients to other services is another example of individual-level public health nursing care.

The recipients of services may also be families, groups, or subpopulations. Health teaching and surveillance are examples of interventions that may be carried out with these larger families, groups, or subpopulations in mind. The identification of high-risk groups within a vulnerable population is a skill of public health nurses. For example, public health nurses create nutrition education programs in schools where obesity is prevalent, or conduct HIV screening for those in prisons.

Finally, public health nurses focus on community-level health problems and interventions. Environmental concerns and disaster response planning are often identified based on community assessments—a unique skill that public health nurses practice. The promotion and establishment of legislation and policies that support desired health outcomes are key interventions, essential to public health nursing.

PROFESSIONAL PARTNERS AND COLLABORATION

Public health nurses partner and collaborate with the population and numerous other groups, including, but not limited to:

- Academic and research institutions

- Businesses and industries

- Community organizations, coalitions, and advocacy groups

- Community service agencies such as schools, law enforcement, urban planning, and emergency response

- Faith-based organizations

- Healthcare providers and facilities

- Legislative, regulatory, and policy-making bodies

- Local, state, and federal public health organizations

- Members of the public health team, such as epidemiologists, social workers, health promotion specialists, nutritionists, environmental health workers, and health educators

By joining together with a common goal of improving population health, public health nurses and these various disciplines and organizations create synergistic practices, learn from one another, and influence population health.

TIERS (LEVELS) OF PUBLIC HEALTH NURSING PRACTICE

The Core Competencies for Public Health Nurses (Quad Council, 2011; hereafter "PHN Core Competencies") are significant for public health nursing. The Quad Council, the leading organizational voice for public health nursing, revised the 2004 PHN Core Competencies document to include three tiers or levels of practice. The revision was done to align the PHN Core Competencies with the revised Core Competencies for Public Health Professionals developed by the Council on Linkages between Academia and Public Health Practice (CoL, 2010). The three tiers or levels of practice differentiate competencies for PHN practice (Quad Council, 2012, p. 2) are:

- Basic or generalist level (Tier 1)

- Specialist or mid-level (Tier 2)

- Executive and/or multisystems level (Tier 3)

The revised PHN Core Competencies (Quad Council, 2011) retain the eight domains from the Council on Linkages competencies:

- Analytic assessment

- Policy development/program planning

- Communication

- Cultural competency

- Community dimensions of practice

- Basic public health sciences

- Financial planning and management

- Leadership and systems thinking

The importance of the revised PHN Core Competencies document is the clear alignment of public health nursing—at all tiers or levels of practice—with the disciplinary view, perspectives, and values of public health professionals.

Tier 2 and Tier 3 PHN Core Competencies (Quad Council, 2012) will inform advanced public health nursing practice. The current context of advanced public health nursing practice, and its fit with other advanced nursing practice specialties, is also significant and worth noting. The advanced nursing practice environment for public health nurses is affected by the *Consensus Model for APRN Regulation* (APRN Joint Dialogue Group, 2008). The APRN model identified the master's-prepared nursing specialties of administration, education, informatics, and public health as specialties that do not provide direct care to individuals, do not require regulation beyond licensure as a registered nurse, and, as such, are not included in the designation of advanced practice registered nurse (APRN). The basis for this decision derives from issues of regulation and licensure that align APRNs with medical models of practice (Kulbok & Ervin, 2012).

The PHN Core Competencies were designed to ensure that public health nursing fit in the domain of public health science. *Public Health Nursing: Scope and Standards of Practice, Second Edition,* also delineates competencies for practice; the ANA competencies, however, are designed to ensure that public health nursing fits in the domain of an ANA-recognized nursing specialty. To assure public health nurses that these two sets of competencies are neither in competition nor burdensome to practice, efforts have been made to align the standards and competencies of this document with the PHN Core Competencies document. The "crosswalk" in Appendix A correlates the Tier 1 competencies with the ANA PHN standards and accompanying competencies.

Influences on Public Health Nursing Practice

There are multiple factors, reports, and other initiatives influencing how public health nurses conceptualize and define the practice of public health nursing in the 21st century.

INSTITUTE OF MEDICINE (IOM) REPORTS

Two IOM reports have been pivotal in shaping public health nursing with regard to public health practice. They include *The Future of the Public's Health in the Twenty-First Century* (IOM, 2003a), which provides direction for defining and creating new approaches in public health practice, education, and research using the ecological model to alter social determinants of health. The companion IOM report, *Who Will Keep the Public Healthy?* (IOM, 2003b) builds on the ecological approach and delineates eight content domains for public health professionals: informatics, genomics, communication, cultural competency, community-based participatory research, policy and law, global health, and ethics. The emphasis in this latter report is on the development of the public health workforce. In terms of nursing in particular, the report *The Future of Nursing: Leading Change, Advancing Health* (IOM, 2011) is a call to action for the health system and nurses. This report responds to the need to assess and transform the nursing profession to emphasize the key role nurses must play in redesigning health care in the United States.

Yet another IOM report, released in March 2012, *Primary Care and Public Health: Exploring Integration to Improve Population Health*, will significantly influence future public health nursing practice. The following statement from the report summary encapsulates implications for PHN practice and population health:

> *Achieving substantial and lasting improvements in population health will require a concerted effort from all of these entities, aligned with a common goal. The integration of primary care and public health could enhance the capacity of both sectors to carry out their respective missions and link with other stakeholders to catalyze a collaborative, intersectoral movement toward improved population health. (p. S-1)*

This IOM report defined *primary care* as "the provision of integrated, accessible healthcare services by clinicians who are accountable for addressing a large majority of personal healthcare needs, developing a sustained partnership with patients, and practicing in the context of family and community" (IOM, 1996, p. 1; 2012, p. S-1). It defined *public health* as "fulfilling society's interest in assuring conditions in which people can be healthy" (IOM, 1988,

p. 140; 2012, p. S-2). The report goes on to describe necessary linkages and partnerships, as well as specific activities in which integration of primary care and public health can be achieved. The language in the 2012 IOM report is consistent with the scope of practice of public health nurses. The timing of this report is strategic with respect to the economics and politics of health care. In addition, the report strongly recommends future funding, enhanced collaboration, and increased willingness of primary care partners in nursing and other disciplines to improve population health. Public health nurses must recognize and seize opportunities for leadership in health promotion and disease prevention to improve population health.

NATIONAL HEALTH INITIATIVES

Several national-level health initiatives influence the practice of public health nursing, as they frame the national priorities for funding and programs concerning health issues. Public health nurses, whether developing new programs or working within existing ones, strive to align their mission and goals with those of national initiatives. Among these are *Healthy People 2020* (U.S. Department of Health and Human Services [DHHS], 2010), the National Prevention Strategy (U.S. DHHS, 2011), and the United States Preventive Services Task Force guide to community preventive services (Agency for Healthcare Research and Quality [AHRQ], 2010).

Healthy People 2020 provides science-based, 10-year national objectives for improving the health of all Americans. It establishes benchmarks and monitors progress over time to measure the impact of prevention activities. The overarching goals of *Healthy People 2020* are to attain high-quality, longer lives free of preventable disease, disability, injury, and premature death. These goals are intended to achieve health equity, eliminate disparities, and improve the health of all groups. *Healthy People 2020* supports the creation of social and physical environments that promote good health for all, while promoting quality of life, healthy development, and healthy behaviors across all life stages.

The National Prevention Strategy presents a framework for prevention and health promotion to improve health in the United States. The National Prevention Strategy is a framework that involves almost every element of life in the promotion of health, from clinical services, to healthy communities, to empowerment and behavior change, to elimination of health disparities. Public health nurses can use this framework as a guide to developing population-based programs, initiatives, and services.

The U.S. Preventive Services Task Force, appointed by the Agency for Healthcare Research and Quality, reviews a broad range of clinical preventive healthcare services and develops evidence-based recommendations for primary care clinicians and health systems. The Task Force oversees the production of *Guide to Community Preventive Services*, also known as the *Community Guide* (AHRQ, 2010), which is a resource for evidence-based recommendations and findings to improve public health. The *Community Guide* provides state-of-the-art systematic reviews that analyze scientific evidence on what works to promote health and prevent disease, injury, and disability. It facilitates assessment of the economic benefits of the interventions found to be effective and identifies critical research gaps.

GLOBAL PUBLIC HEALTH NURSING INITIATIVES

The global nature of health raises many opportunities and challenges for public health nursing, including the global burden of disease; the health implications of migration, travel, and displacement; the social and environmental determinants of health; and health care in low-resource settings. Public health nurses contribute to improving population health in both domestic and international settings through bidirectional efforts. They provide services, lead initiatives, and develop health systems and policies aimed at achieving national goals as well as the health-related targets of the internationally agreed-upon United Nations Development Program's Millennium Development Goals (MDGs).

Several World Health Assembly (WHA) resolutions (WHA 42.27, WHA 45.5, WHA 49.1, WHA 54.12) demonstrate the importance of nursing services to achieve better health for all communities. WHA 54.12 states that "nurses and midwives[1] play a crucial and cost-effective role in reducing excess mortality, morbidity, and disability and in promoting healthy lifestyles." Most recently, the Department of Human Resources for Health of the World Health Organization (WHO) produced the *Strategic Directions for Strengthening Nursing and Midwifery Services 2011–2015* document (WHO, 2012), which provides a framework for collaborative action to improve health outcomes through the provision of competent, culturally sensitive, evidence-based nursing and midwifery services.

---

[1] In the context of international nursing, nurses and midwives are synonymous, and "midwives" are not necessarily advanced practice registered nurses as in the United States. For consistency with international health agency text, the terms *midwives* and *midwifery* are preserved in this section, though not connoting that public health nurses in the United States are necessarily midwives.

Several formal organizational relationships support public health nursing practice in the global context, including the WHO Nursing and Midwifery Office, the Global Advisory Group in Nursing and Midwifery, and the Global Network of WHO Collaborating Centers in Nursing and Midwifery Development. The International Council of Nurses, International Confederation of Midwives, and Sigma Theta Tau International Honor Society of Nursing are examples of international organizations that support global public health nurses in achieving both national health goals and health-related targets of the MDGs.

ETHICAL CONSIDERATIONS

Public health nurses are bound by the ethical provisions for all nurses explicit in *Code of Ethics for Nurses with Interpretive Statements* (ANA, 2001), *Principles of Ethical Practice of Public Health* (Public Health Leadership Society, 2002), and *Environmental Health Principles and Recommendations for Public Health Nursing* (APHA, 2006). Ethical practice requires invoking strategies to address multiple determinants of health, health disparity, health promotion, and health policy to improve health communication at all levels of health-related engagement (Baur, 2010). In working with populations, public health nurses must acknowledge the right of the population to have access to the necessary information and opportunities for dialogue in order to make informed decisions without coercion.

The purpose of public health nursing science is to enhance the health of populations. Public health nurses must recognize and establish their professional practice in accordance with the populations' rights and with a particular concern for social justice. This includes using the "precautionary principle" to guide practice and engage in preventive actions in the face of uncertainty, and exploring a wide range of alternatives to potentially harmful actions, as well as promoting increased public participation in decision-making (Raffensberger & Tickner, 1998). In addition, when participating in activities where decisions are made that have an impact on health, public health nurses are obligated to assure that ethical issues are addressed as part of the decision-making process. Public health nurses should also be represented on ethics bodies that make decisions affecting the rights of the population and public health nurses.

Advocacy focused on public health is another important facet of public health nursing that requires ethical consideration, specifically related to the contexts of healthcare reform and changing demographics of the U.S. population. The healthcare system is ever-evolving on a policy and legislative level; therefore, public health nurses have the obligation to educate and inform populations to guarantee access to health care all. This includes political activism on behalf of vulnerable populations and ensuring that health care is delivered in an equitable, fair, and competent manner, regardless of health insurance status or the presence of illness.

Yet another consideration is that of the changing demographics of the United States. According to the U.S. Census Bureau, the majority of the U.S. population will be composed of traditionally underrepresented ethnic minorities by 2050. As of the 2010 census, Latinos have surpassed African Americans as the largest minority group in the United States. These changes in demographics call for an increased awareness of barriers to health care and education of healthcare professionals in cultural competency and language access in health care. These issues are also closely tied to healthcare reform, as minorities are more likely than Caucasian Americans to be in poor health, have low income, and be uninsured.

Advances in scientific, medical, and healthcare technologies create ethical and legal questions that must be addressed while respecting the diverse beliefs, cultures, and values present in the populations served. The widespread availability and use of social networking and devices enabled with Internet access provide unique opportunities for educating individuals and families within populations on ways to protect, promote, and enhance their own health. However, they also require constant vigilance, due to their ability to transmit data, pictures, and other information that is "protected," to avoid breaches of privacy and consequent damage to trust in the individual public health nurse, the profession, and public health in general. The need to receive or share information concerning an individual's health in order to protect the health of the public creates a unique set of ethical issues for public health nurses. With the transition to electronic health records, the establishment of health information exchanges, and implementation of other components of the HITECH Act, sharing of data for public health purposes becomes much easier. However, the implementation of these systems to promote safety and quality of care must be done with a specific focus on the privacy and security of this information. Likewise, the use of genomics in researching etiology and treatment of disease to prevent morbidity and mortality must be done with beneficence, without disenfranchising or limiting access to care for certain populations.

Health literacy, an ethical dimension of every registered nurse's practice, is particularly important for public health nurses. Health literacy is defined as "[t]he degree to which individuals have the capacity to obtain, process, and understand basic health information and services needed to make appropriate health decisions" (IOM, 2004; U.S. DHHS, 2000). Poor health literacy is pervasive, vaguely understood, and contributes to morbidity and sometimes death in vulnerable populations.

Vulnerable populations with lower health literacy scores include those with educational levels of less than a high school diploma, lower socioeconomic levels, some ethnic minorities, and those with limited English proficiency. In a 2003 national adult health literacy survey (Kutner, Greenberg, Jin, & Paulsen, 2006), up to 30% of uninsured adults or those on Medicare or Medicaid had poor health literacy skills. Poor health literacy negatively influences individual communication (patient–provider communication, clinical interactions, and prescription usage) and population-level outreach (understanding prevention guidelines and navigating healthcare systems).

Education and Preparation

The landscape of higher education in nursing has changed during the past decade. The clinical nurse leader (CNL), a generalist master's degree, and the doctor of nursing practice (DNP) degree, a specialized practice doctorate, provide new options for educational advancement in the profession of nursing. As reflected in the *Tier 1 Competencies for Public Health Nursing* (Quad Council, 2012), the educational credentials for entry into public health nursing practice are the baccalaureate degree in nursing or the CNL generalist master's. A master of science in nursing (MSN), master of public health (MPH), a joint MSN/MPH, or a doctorate degree (i.e., doctor of philosophy [PhD], doctor of nursing practice [DNP], doctor of public health [DrPH]), is assumed for the public health nurse specialist with a specific focus in population health. Educational preparation at the specialty MSN or DNP level best prepares public health nurses to function in the specialty role as advanced public health nurses (see discussion later in this section). Associate-degree and diploma-prepared registered nurses, and licensed practical nurses, might appropriately practice in some public health settings providing care for individuals or families, but not with populations.

In the accompanying standards of practice, the term *advanced public health nurse* is used to describe the additional expectations of master's-prepared public health nurses who function at the advanced nursing practice level in population health, as delineated in the CCPHN Tier 2 and Tier 3 competencies. The advanced public health nurse must meet all of the educational and practice criteria required for both generalist and specialist public health nursing practice. Core content areas for advanced public health nursing include advanced nursing practice, social and behavioral sciences, population-centered nursing theory and practice, interdisciplinary practice, leadership, systems thinking, biostatistics, epidemiology, environmental health sciences, health policy and management, public health informatics, genomics, health communication, cultural competence, community-based participatory research, global health, policy and law, and public health ethics (Levin, Cary, Kulbok, Leffers, Molle, & Polivka, 2008). Additional scope and standards documents might apply to public health nurses working in other nursing specialties or roles, such as administration, corrections, or school health.

Many specialist public health nursing practice roles require knowledge, skills, and abilities that necessitate a practice-focused or a research-focused doctoral degree. Multiple venues for pursuing doctoral-level education exist, and program selection may depend on the role the public health nurse holds or wishes to hold (e.g., advanced clinical practice or research focus, interdisciplinary public health, informatics, epidemiology, ethics). The individual public health nurse pursuing a DNP degree or the research doctorate (e.g., doctor of philosophy [PhD]) needs to assure that population health is a central component of the selected course of study.

All public health nurses are expected to be lifelong learners. This means they actively engage in a process of self-assessment to review their current knowledge, skills, and abilities and to identify areas for further development. Such professional development may include enrollment in a formal academic program or participation in continuing education. Specialty certification in public health nursing is available from the American Nurses Credentialing Center (ANCC): these include, for example, the advanced public health nurse (APHN-BC) or the public health nursing clinical nurse specialist (PHCNS-BC) certifications. The PHCNS-BC credential is available for master's-prepared public health nurses who have also taken courses in pathophysiology, pharmacology, and physical assessment. In addition, specialty certification in public health is available from the National Board of Public Health Examiners for nurses and other public health professionals who have earned an MPH degree; an example is the certificate of public health (CPH).

Issues and Trends in Public Health Nursing

NECESSARY KNOWLEDGE BASE FOR PUBLIC HEALTH NURSING

Public health nurses must be prepared to effect positive changes at the population level by tailoring intervention strategies and shaping environments with other disciplines and the community to support health for individuals, families, groups, communities, and populations. This is especially important as more non-communicable diseases, which are related to behavioral choices (e.g., nicotine addiction, obesity), become heightened population health threats. Awareness, knowledge, and leadership skills are integral to public health nursing practice so that the practitioner can influence policy, prevention programs, social marketing strategies, and surveillance evaluation. Public health nursing practice requires the expertise to overcome the impact of misinformation and social commercial marketing that encourage populations to make poor health choices.

Public health nurses require competency in health and social policy development. Severe economic conditions worldwide create immense challenges for societies, both industrial and developing, to maintain and improve the health and wellness of their citizens. Compounding these challenges are global population changes, including climate change, the increasing global census, and increased life expectancy. Public health nurses must be attuned to changes in health, economic, and political policies that affect populations on the local, state, federal, and international levels. They are involved in developing and monitoring regulatory strategies related to current or future healthcare laws, and active in integrating health policy and economics into all levels of public health nursing education and practice. As local, state, federal, and international budgets related to the provision of healthcare services shrink and public scrutiny increases, public health nurses evaluate the outcomes of community and population interventions to fully articulate the return on investment.

Monitoring shifts in health policy includes understanding the development of structural systems and evolving models of healthcare delivery and reimbursement. These models include patient-centered healthcare programs, nontraditional community learning experiences (e.g., clinics located in drugstores or truck stops; engagement of homeless populations to assess and provide interventions), and changes in Medicare and Medicaid delivery systems. Other models that will influence public health systems include accountable care organizations, accreditation programs, transitional care models, and value-based purchasing. These changes will escalate with the implementation of the Affordable Care Act.

PUBLIC HEALTH DEPARTMENT ACCREDITATION

Over the past several years, there has been an increasing amount of interest in developing performance standards linked to an accreditation process for governmental public health departments in the United States. This evolution will require public health nurses, particularly at the advanced level, to focus on outcomes measurement and tools to improve quality in order to meet accreditation standards.

The foundation of this movement was rooted in Institute of Medicine reports in 1988 and 2003, which described the governmental public health infrastructure as being in disarray. However, these reports also noted the importance of public health as the "backbone" of a community. After studying the issue carefully, the Robert Wood Johnson Foundation and the Centers for Disease Control and Prevention funded the establishment of a national voluntary public health department accreditation program.

The Public Health Accreditation Board (PHAB) was created to serve as the national body for the development and implementation of accreditation for state, local, tribal, and territorial health departments. The development of national public health accreditation has involved, and is supported by, public health leaders and practitioners from the national, tribal, state, and local levels. National public health accreditation, as administered by the PHAB, is based on a goal of improving and protecting the health of the public by advancing the quality and performance of state, local, tribal, and territorial public health departments. Accreditation of the health department is one important step on the journey to creating a culture of quality improvement in public health.

Deliberately designed to be nonregulatory in its approach, PHAB's accreditation process includes:

- The measurement of health department performance against a set of nationally recognized, practice-focused, and evidence-based standards

- The issuance of recognition of achievement of accreditation within a specified time frame by a nationally recognized entity

- The continual development, revision, and distribution of public health standards

The PHAB deployed a framework of 10 essential public health services in developing its accreditation standards and measures (PHAB, 2011). Two domains were added around which health departments are peer-reviewed, as follows:

- Maintain administrative and management capacity

- Build a strong and effective relationship with governing entity

DIGITAL TECHNOLOGY IN COMMUNICATION AND INFORMATION USE AND MANAGEMENT

Dramatic paradigm shifts in communication and electronic recordkeeping impact the way people communicate, learn, live, and work. Public health nurses will also use tools such as health impact assessment (HIA) for community monitoring of environmental indicators affecting health. Other uses of technology include enlargement of national and global "virtual" meetings, collaboration, and education; increased online "asynchronous" learning; leadership training and engagement; and telehealth care.

Summary of the Scope of Public Health Nursing Practice

Population health is the dynamic synthesis of the outcomes of many collaborative strategies implemented by public health nurses, community members, intersectoral health professionals, and other key stakeholders. As influences on the health of the public encompass global communities, public health nursing practice becomes increasingly complex. Deeper understanding of concepts of complexity, community participatory approaches, informatics, and other emerging theories and methodologies will allow public health nurses to practice more effectively. Future public health nurses will create dynamic micro- and macro-linkages between individuals and populations, explore past and current healthcare issues and trends in order to develop innovative population health strategies, and engage in constructing the context for policy development to support relationships that promote the achievement of population health. The practice of public health nursing is an established nursing specialty and requires expanded scientific inquiry and research to continue practice improvement. Public health nurses must concentrate on building and merging the nursing, social, and public health sciences to create innovative approaches that reflect the complexity and dynamic nature of health care and population health.

As care shifts from acute settings to community settings, a shift in the image of public health nursing must also occur. The brand and image of public health nursing as "specialists" who care for populations should be endorsed. Public health nurses must excel in building their specialist image and clarifying their roles within the nursing profession and beyond, with the public. This clarification is essential to increase collaboration with nursing colleagues, primary care providers, and the public. The development of innovative ways of recruiting and mentoring public health nurses will assist in ensuring that the PHN workforce is sufficient to meet the new paradigm of health promotion and wellness as a framework for healthcare systems.

Standards of Professional Public Health Nursing Practice

Significance of Standards

The Standards of Professional Nursing Practice are authoritative statements of the duties that all registered nurses, regardless of role, population, or specialty, are expected to perform competently. The standards published herein may be utilized as evidence of the standard of care, with the understanding that application of the standards is context dependent. The standards are subject to change with the dynamics of the nursing profession, as new patterns of professional practice are developed and accepted by the nursing profession and the public. In addition, specific conditions and clinical circumstances may also affect the application of the standards at a given time (e.g., during a natural disaster). The standards are subject to formal, periodic review and revision.

The competencies that accompany each standard may be evidence of compliance with the corresponding standard. The list of competencies is not exhaustive. Whether a particular standard or competency applies depends upon the circumstances.

As a specialty recognized by the American Nurses Association, public health nursing conforms its standards to the model document, *Nursing: Scope and Standards of Practice, Second Edition* (ANA, 2010). The standard language is identical to that of the model document, yet the competencies differ, reflecting public health nursing's demonstration of how practice is specialized.

Standards of Practice for Public Health Nursing

Standard 1. Assessment

The public health nurse collects comprehensive data pertinent to the health status of populations.

COMPETENCIES

The public health nurse:

- Collects comprehensive, multisource data in a systematic and ongoing process related to the health of the population or specific subpopulation, including assets, resources, and multiple determinants of health.

- Partners with the population and other key stakeholders in the assessment process.

- Elicits the population's unique beliefs, needs, and values, and includes health literacy level in the assessment.

- Identifies barriers and limitations (e.g., cultural power, health literacy, socioeconomic inequities) to effective communication and comprehensive data collection.

- Prioritizes assessment based on immediate, urgent, or anticipated risk or need in geographic areas or in populations.

- Uses evidence-based principles, models, and tools of epidemiology, demography, and biostatistics, as well as social, behavioral, and natural and applied sciences to structure data collection.

- Synthesizes data to identify and interpret trends and deviations from expected health patterns in the population.

- Uses an ecological perspective in health assessment.

- Applies ethical, legal, and privacy guidelines and policies to the collection, maintenance, use, and dissemination of data and information.

- Identifies variables that measure public health and public health conditions.

- Identifies sources of public health data and information.

- Analyzes data using evidence-based models and problem-solving techniques from nursing, public health, and other disciplines.

- Documents assessment data in a retrievable format and in terms that are understandable to all involved in the process.

ADDITIONAL COMPETENCIES FOR THE ADVANCED PUBLIC HEALTH NURSE

The advanced public health nurse:

- Gathers data from multiple, interdisciplinary sources using appropriate methods to augment and/or verify population-focused data.

- Partners with populations, health professionals, and other stakeholders to attach meaning to collected data.

- Synthesizes qualitative and quantitative data during data analysis for a comprehensive population assessment.

- Consults with other public health professionals, the population, the interdisciplinary team, and other stakeholders in the design, management, and evaluation of the data system that focuses on population assets, needs, and concerns.

Standard 2. Population Diagnosis and Priorities

The public health nurse analyzes the assessment data to determine the diagnoses or issues.

COMPETENCIES

The public health nurse:

- Derives comprehensive population diagnoses and priorities based on assessment data.

- Validates the diagnoses or concerns with the population and local, state, and federal public health agencies and organizations.

- Identifies actual or potential risks to the population's health and safety, as well as barriers to health, which may include, but are not limited to, interpersonal, systematic, or environmental circumstances.

- Documents diagnoses or concerns in a manner that facilitates population involvement in the determination of the plan and its expected outcomes.

ADDITIONAL COMPETENCIES FOR THE ADVANCED PUBLIC HEALTH NURSE

The advanced public health nurse:

- Utilizes complex data and information obtained during sociocultural, demographic, health status and health risk, geographic, environmental, and other nursing and public health diagnostic processes to identify population health assets, needs, and risks.

- Systematically analyzes relevant population data, incorporating scientific evidence and principles, as well as community input, in formulating population-focused diagnoses and in setting priorities.

- Assists staff and stakeholders in developing and maintaining competence in the population diagnosis process.

Standard 3. Outcomes Identification

The public health nurse identifies expected outcomes for a plan specific to the population or situation.

COMPETENCIES

The public health nurse:

- Involves the population, other professionals, organizations, and stakeholders in formulating expected outcomes.

- Derives culturally appropriate expected outcomes from the diagnoses.

- Considers population beliefs and values, benefits and risks, costs, current scientific evidence, current social policies, and own expertise when formulating expected outcomes.

- Incorporates knowledge of available resources; environmental factors and events; ethical, legal, and privacy considerations; and time estimates in defining expected outcomes.

- Develops expected outcomes that reflect a long-term commitment to enhancing population assets and meeting needs and concerns.

- Modifies expected outcomes based on changes in the status of the population needs or concerns and the availability of resources.

- Documents expected outcomes as measurable objectives using language that is understandable to all involved entities.

ADDITIONAL COMPETENCIES FOR THE ADVANCED PUBLIC HEALTH NURSE

The advanced public health nurse:

- Involves interprofessional partners in identifying expected outcomes that incorporate scientific evidence and are achievable through implementation of evidence-based practices.

- Incorporates factors such as continuity and consistency of the services; cost-effectiveness; satisfaction of stakeholders, the population, and the organization; and resolution of health concerns into measurable outcomes.

- Differentiates outcomes that require individual/family or community interventions from those that require system-level interventions.

Standard 4. Planning

The public health nurse develops a plan that prescribes strategies and alternatives to attain expected outcomes.

COMPETENCIES

The public health nurse:

- Contributes to the development of population-focused plans for health-related services or programs based on an assessment and prioritization of determinants of health, health assets, concerns, needs, and risks.

- Establishes plans that reflect scientific evidence, communication and learning principles, and cultural competence, and sets priorities and timelines that address the population needs.

- Incorporates evidence-based strategies that address the identified diagnoses, concerns, or needs, including, but not limited to:

  - Promotion, improvement, and restoration of health

  - Prevention of illness, injury, or disease

  - Alleviation of suffering

  - Emergency preparedness and response

- Includes population-focused strategies for health and wholeness across the lifespan.

- Partners with members of the identified population, health professionals, coalitions, organizations, and other stakeholders in determining roles within the planning processes.

- Applies current policies, regulations, standards, and statutes in the planning process.

- Modifies the plan according to an ongoing assessment of population outcomes.

- Uses an ecological perspective in planning.

- Documents the plan using language that is culturally sensitive and at an appropriate reading level that can be understood by all participants.

- Integrates current and emerging trends and research in nursing and public health-related fields in the planning process.

- Provides for continuity within and across programs and services.

ADDITIONAL COMPETENCIES FOR THE ADVANCED PUBLIC HEALTH NURSE

The advanced public health nurse:

- Applies assessment, implementation, and evaluation strategies within the plan to reflect current evidence, including data, research, literature, and expert nursing and public health knowledge.

- Designs appropriate strategies and alternatives with community and professional partners to meet the complex needs of at-risk populations.

- Incorporates population beliefs and values with community and professional partners in the planning process.

- Leads other public health nurses and the multisector team in the use of principles of planning for population-focused programs and services.

- Contributes to the development and continuous improvement of organizational systems that support the planning process.

- Participates in the integration of fiscal, human, material, population, and scientific resources to enhance and complete the planning process for programs or services.

Standard 5. Implementation

The public health nurse implements the identified plan.

COMPETENCIES

The public health nurse:

- Partners with individuals, families, groups, and communities to implement the plan in a safe, realistic, and timely manner in collaboration with the multisector team.

- Applies evidence-based strategies, activities, and outcome measures, including opportunities for ongoing advocacy and coalition building, in the implementation of a plan that is specific to the population assets, collaborative needs, resources, and concerns with measured outcomes.

- Provides holistic care that addresses the needs of populations across the lifespan.

- Incorporates systems and population resources during implementation of the plan.

- Applies appropriate knowledge of cultural diversity and major health problems in implementing the plan.

- Integrates the ecological perspective into implementation of the plan.

- Monitors implementation of the plan, including processes, resource utilization, and outcome measures.

- Collaborates with others from diverse backgrounds to implement and integrate the plan.

- Accommodates different styles of communication used by the population and other providers and stakeholders.

- Integrates traditional and complementary healthcare practices as appropriate.

- Documents implementation of the plan, lessons learned, modifications, progress, and outcomes.

- Uses technology to measure, record, and retrieve data; implement the nursing process; and enhance nursing practice.

ADDITIONAL COMPETENCIES FOR THE ADVANCED
PUBLIC HEALTH NURSE

The advanced public health nurse:

- Interprets surveillance data related to the plan and population health status.

- Incorporates new knowledge and strategies into action plans to enhance implementation.

- Designs solutions to internal and external barriers or challenges that may affect implementation of the plan.

- Modifies the plan based on appropriate health behavior change theory, new knowledge, population response, or other relevant factors to achieve expected outcomes.

- Advocates for needed resources for implementation of the plan with the subject population.

- Champions new and ongoing collaborative relationships to implement the plan.

- Assures appropriate dissemination of the plan and its outcomes to provide transparency of accomplishments, challenges, and efforts.

Standard 5A. Coordination of Care

The public health nurse coordinates care delivery.

COMPETENCIES

The public health nurse:

- Promotes policies, programs, and services for attainment of the expected outcome.

- Incorporates individual and/or family care management, to include broad community coordination of public health services.

- Conducts surveillance, case finding, and other reporting functions with health professionals and other stakeholders.

- Connects populations with needed services.

- Implements follow-up on coordination of referrals and appropriate interventions as a member of the public health and nursing team.

- Documents coordination of care.

- Applies best practices for coordination to attain effective public health nursing care.

ADDITIONAL COMPETENCIES FOR THE ADVANCED PUBLIC HEALTH NURSE

The advanced public health nurse:

- Provides leadership for the coordination of interprofessional health care for integrated programs, services, and public policy, including with intersectoral providers.

- Synthesizes data and information to prescribe necessary system and community support measures.

Standard 5B. Health Teaching and Health Promotion

The public health nurse employs multiple strategies to promote health and a safe environment.

COMPETENCIES

The public health nurse:

- Includes appropriate health education in the planning and implementation of programs and services for populations, including, but not limited to:

  - Available resources

  - Developmental needs

  - Healthy lifestyle choices and behaviors

  - Health promotion, disease prevention, and risk-reduction strategies

  - Multiple determinants of health

- Selects teaching and learning methods using appropriate health literacy strategies and focused on the objectives and resources identified by the population.

- Uses evidence-based health promotion and health education models and methods appropriate to the situation and the population's attitudes, beliefs, culture, and values; developmental level; learning needs; readiness and ability to learn; language preference; health practices; socioeconomic status; and spirituality.

- Provides anticipatory guidance to individuals, families, groups, and communities to promote health and prevent or reduce the risk of health problems.

- Provides individuals, families, groups, communities, and populations with information about intended effects and potential adverse effects of proposed policies, programs, and services.

- Seeks opportunities for feedback and evaluation of the effectiveness of the strategies used.

- Uses appropriate information technology to deliver health promotion and disease prevention information.

- Uses an ecological perspective and knowledge of the multiple determinants of health to work effectively with diverse populations.

- Addresses factors contributing to cultural diversity.

ADDITIONAL COMPETENCIES FOR THE ADVANCED PUBLIC HEALTH NURSE

The advanced public health nurse:

- Synthesizes empirical evidence on risk behaviors, behavior change theories, epidemiology, health communication models, learning theories, motivational theories, and other related theories and frameworks when designing health education information and health promotion programs.

- Evaluates health information resources for accuracy, clarity, and readability to help targeted populations access quality health information.

- Incorporates comparative effectiveness research recommendations into health education and health promotion strategies.

- Provides leadership to nursing and other health professionals in planning evidence-based health promotion programs and services based upon current assessments, identification of population-specific and prioritized needs, understanding of policy issues, and appropriate planning and evaluation strategies.

- Engages advocacy groups and consumer alliances, as appropriate, in health education and health promotion activities.

- Modifies existing health education and health promotion programs based on feedback from participants, providers, health professionals, and other stakeholders.

Standard 5C. Consultation

The public health nurse provides consultation to influence the identified plan, enhance the abilities of others, and effect change.

COMPETENCIES

The public health nurse:

- Partners with community organizations and groups to facilitate participation in programs and services.

- Provides testimony and professional opinion on programs, policies, and service delivery with populations.

- Communicates effectively with constituent groups during consultation, using a variety of media.

- Documents the scope and effectiveness of consultation activities provided to community populations.

ADDITIONAL COMPETENCIES FOR THE ADVANCED PUBLIC HEALTH NURSE

The advanced public health nurse:

- Synthesizes data from local, state, federal, and other sources, in consultation with community and other public health system stakeholders.

- Provides expert testimony at the local, state, and federal levels on program and service delivery to at-risk populations.

- Communicates consultation recommendations.

- Generates proposals and reports in support of needed programs and services.

Standard 5D. Prescriptive Authority

Not applicable

Standard 5E. Regulatory Activities

The public health nurse participates in applications of public health laws, regulations, and policies.

COMPETENCIES

The public health nurse:

- Describes the structure, function, and jurisdictional authority of the organizational units within local, tribal, state, and federal public health agencies and their impacts on individuals, families, and groups within a population.

- Educates affected populations on the development and application of relevant laws, regulations, and policies.

- Supports public health policies, programs, and resources.

- Completes monitoring and inspection activities for regulated entities.

- Collects specific information about situations that are reported to public health officials to inform policy decisions.

- Assists with addressing noncompliance with laws, regulations, and policies.

- Contributes in emergency preparedness and response efforts, including the receipt and use of the strategic national stockpile.

- Contributes to the intersectoral team to implement public health regulatory requirements such as case identification, mandatory reporting, and program management.

ADDITIONAL COMPETENCIES FOR THE ADVANCED
PUBLIC HEALTH NURSE

The advanced public health nurse:

- Collaborates in the development of public health laws, regulations, and policies.

- With other public health professionals, designs compliance and reporting systems related to laws, regulations, and policies.

- Monitors compliance and reporting systems for quality and appropriate use of resources.

- Analyzes data and compiles reports for public health officials and other decision-makers as required by laws, regulations, and policies.

Standard 6. Evaluation

The public health nurse evaluates progress toward attainment of outcomes.

COMPETENCIES

The public health nurse:

- Conducts a systematic, ongoing, and criterion-based evaluation of program and service outcomes in relation to the recommended program plan and the indicated timeline.

- Collaborates with the target population and other key stakeholders involved in the evaluation process.

- Collects data systematically, applying epidemiological and scientific methods to determine the effectiveness of public health nursing interventions on policies, programs, and services.

- Uses information technology to understand the impact of multiple determinants of health.

- Uses ongoing assessment data to identify gaps and redundancies, and to revise plans, interventions, and activities as needed.

- Disseminates the evaluation results to the population and other stakeholders in accordance with state and federal laws and regulations, as appropriate.

- Participates in evaluation by monitoring and assuring appropriate use of programs and services to minimize unnecessary burden on the population.

- Documents the results of the evaluation, including changes or recommendations to enhance effectiveness of programs, services, and interventions.

ADDITIONAL COMPETENCIES FOR THE ADVANCED PUBLIC HEALTH NURSE

The advanced public health nurse:

- Designs an evaluation plan with other public health experts and with population representatives and other stakeholders.

- Evaluates the accuracy of the assessed population health need or problem and the effectiveness of the plan and other variables in relationship to expected and unexpected outcomes.

- Synthesizes the results of the evaluation analyses to determine the effect of the program plan on populations, organizations, and other key stakeholder groups.

- Adapts the evaluation plan for policies, programs, or services, as appropriate.

- Uses the results of the evaluation analyses to recommend or make changes, including policy, procedure, program, or service revision, as appropriate.

Standards of Professional Performance for Public Health Nursing

Standard 7. Ethics

The public health nurse practices ethically.

COMPETENCIES

The public health nurse:

- Applies *Code of Ethics for Nurses with Interpretive Statements* (ANA, 2001) to guide public health nursing practice.

- Adheres to the *Principles of Ethical Practice of Public Health* (Public Health Leadership Society, 2002) and principles of social justice to achieve the greater good of the whole.

- Delivers programs and services in a manner that preserves, promotes, and protects the autonomy, beliefs, dignity, values, and rights of individuals, communities, and populations.

- Applies ethical standards in advocating for the health of populations and social policy.

- Maintains individual confidentiality within legal and regulatory parameters.

- Assists populations, communities, and individuals in developing skills in self-determination and informed decision-making.

- Maintains professional relationships and boundaries with individuals, families, and groups within the population while delivering public health services and programs.

- Demonstrates a commitment to resolving social and environmental issues and barriers to healthy living conditions that contribute to health inequities.

- Contributes to resolving ethical issues involving colleagues, community groups, systems, and other stakeholders.

- Reports activities that are inconsistent with accepted standards of practice, illegal, unethical, or reflective of impaired practice.

- Challenges public health practices that jeopardize safety or quality improvement.

ADDITIONAL COMPETENCIES FOR THE ADVANCED PUBLIC HEALTH NURSE

The advanced public health nurse:

- Informs populations and communities of the benefits, outcomes, and risks of policies, programs, and services.

- Informs administrators, stakeholders, and/or other providers of the benefits, outcomes, and risks of policies, programs, and services, and related decisions that affect the delivery of health-related services.

- Partners with multisector teams to address ethical benefits, outcomes, and risks of policies, programs, and services.

- Promotes solutions to social and environmental issues and barriers to healthy living conditions.

Standard 8. Education

The public health nurse attains knowledge and competence that reflect current nursing practice.

COMPETENCIES

The public health nurse:

- Participates in ongoing educational activities related to appropriate nursing and public health knowledge and professional issues.

- Demonstrates a commitment to lifelong learning through self-reflection and inquiry to address learning and personal growth needs.

- Seeks experiences that reflect current practice to maintain knowledge, skills, abilities, and judgment in the implementation of policies, programs, and services for populations.

- Describes how individual, family, group, and community-focused programs contribute to meeting the core public health foundations and the 10 essential public health services.

- Acquires knowledge and skills, including those relate to technology, appropriate to the public health nursing role, specialty, setting, or situation.

- Describes the historical foundation of public health and public health nursing.

- Seeks formal and independent learning experiences to develop and maintain skills and knowledge related to population health.

- Identifies learning needs based on nursing and public health knowledge, the various roles the nurse may assume, and the changing needs of the population.

- Identifies changes in the statutory requirements for the practice of nursing and public health.

- Participates in formal or informal consultations to address issues in public health nursing practice and education.

- Shares educational experiences, findings, and ideas with peers.

■ Contributes to a work environment conducive to the education of healthcare professionals.

■ Maintains professional records that provide evidence of competence and lifelong learning.

ADDITIONAL COMPETENCIES FOR THE ADVANCED PUBLIC HEALTH NURSE

The advanced public health nurse:

■ Uses current research findings and other evidence to expand nursing and public health knowledge, skills, abilities, and judgment to enhance role performance and increase knowledge of professional issues.

Standard 9. Evidence-Based Practice and Research

The public health nurse integrates evidence and research findings into practice.

COMPETENCIES

The public health nurse:

- Utilizes the best current evidence, including nursing and public health research findings, to guide practice, policy, and service delivery decisions.

- Participates in the formulation of evidence-based practice through research activities, as appropriate to education level and position. Such activities may include:

  - Engaging in outcomes research focusing on multiple determinants of health with communities and partners

  - Identifying community and professional opportunities suitable for public health nursing research

  - Participating in recruitment efforts and data collection

  - Participating in agency, organization, or population-focused research committees, programs, and/or institutional review boards

  - Implementing research protocols

  - Critically analyzing and interpreting research for application to population-focused practice

  - Applying nursing, public health, and social science research findings and systems theory in the development of policies, programs, and services to promote population health

  - Incorporating research as a basis for learning

- Facilitates involvement of communities, populations, organizations, and other stakeholder groups in a participatory research process.

- Shares research activities and/or findings with colleagues and community stakeholders.

- Contributes effectively as a member of a community-based participatory research (CBPR) team.

ADDITIONAL COMPETENCIES FOR THE ADVANCED
PUBLIC HEALTH NURSE

The advanced public health nurse:

- Advocates for access to health sciences literature to enable evidence-based practice.

- Contributes to nursing, public health, and social science knowledge by conducting or synthesizing evidence that discovers, examines, and evaluates current practice, theories, models, criteria, and creative approaches to improve healthcare systems and population health outcomes.

- Integrates best current evidence with professional expertise and community/stakeholder preferences and values for improvement in healthcare systems and population health.

- Promotes research and scientific inquiry in the practice environment.

- Disseminates current evidence through presentations, publications, consultations, and use of other media.

Standard 10. Quality of Practice

The public health nurse contributes to quality nursing practice.

COMPETENCIES

The public health nurse:

- Demonstrates quality by documenting the application of the nursing process in a responsible, accountable, and ethical manner.

- Implements new knowledge and quality improvement activities to initiate changes in practice and the delivery of care of populations.

- Uses creativity and innovation to enhance practice.

- Participates in quality improvement. Activities may include:

  - Identifying aspects of practice important for quality monitoring

  - Using evidence-based indicators to monitor the quality and effectiveness of nursing practice

  - Collecting data to monitor practice, including acceptability, accessibility, availability, and quality effectiveness of policies, programs, and services

  - Analyzing the data to identify opportunities for improving nursing practice and/or population outcomes

  - Formulating recommendations to improve nursing practice and/or population outcomes

  - Implementing activities to enhance the quality of nursing practice and/or population outcomes

  - Participating in and/or leading efforts with the population, other professionals, organizations, and other stakeholders to evaluate policies, programs, and services

  - Participating in and/or leading efforts to reduce costs and unnecessary duplication

  - Identifying opportunities for improvement in day-to-day work routines, in order to address process inefficiencies

- Analyzing factors related to accessibility of services, population safety, and program effectiveness

- Analyzing organization and program processes and systems for barriers to accessibility to services, population safety, program effectiveness, and quality

- Implementing processes to remove or reduce barriers and to enhance assets within programs and organizational systems

- Documents the delivery of programs and services in ways that reflect the quality measures.

ADDITIONAL COMPETENCIES FOR THE ADVANCED PUBLIC HEALTH NURSE

The advanced public health nurse:

- Provides leadership in the design and implementation of quality improvements.

- Designs innovations to effect change in policies, programs, and services based on existing evidence.

- Evaluates the practice environment and quality of nursing care rendered in relation to existing evidence.

- Identifies opportunities for the generation and use of research to enhance the evidence base for public health nursing practice.

- Obtains and maintains professional certification if it is available in the area of expertise.

- Uses the results of quality improvement to initiate changes in public health nursing practice and in programs, policies, and public health systems.

Standard 11. Communication

The public health nurse communicates effectively in a variety of formats in all areas of practice.

COMPETENCIES

The public health nurse:

- Assesses communication format preferences of individuals, families, groups, communities, populations, and interprofessional colleagues.

- Incorporates evidence-based communication techniques, including collaborative and guiding skills, negotiation and conflict resolution, and knowledge of health literacy, to optimize health outcomes and produce effective relationships with individuals, families, groups, communities, populations, and professionals.

- Seeks continuous improvement of individual communication styles using evidence-based communication principles.

- Communicates in written, oral, and electronic modes in a culturally relevant, timely, and legally and ethically responsible manner.

- Translates information across intersectoral partners to ensure accurate and evidence-based communication.

- Conveys information to individuals, families, groups, communities, populations, and interprofessional colleagues in communication formats that promote accuracy, evidence-based practice, and awareness of health literacy.

- Communicates observations and concerns to appropriate decision-making personnel related to population-level hazards and errors in programs, services, and the practice environment.

- Maintains communication with other providers throughout the healthcare system to optimize experiences associated with referrals and transitions in care.

- Modifies practice when necessary to promote positive interaction between individuals, families, groups, and communities; care providers; and technology in the delivery of programs and services.

- Contributes own professional perspective in discussions with the interprofessional team and intersectoral partners.

ADDITIONAL COMPETENCIES FOR THE ADVANCED PUBLIC HEALTH NURSE

The advanced public health nurse:

- Integrates health literacy principles into communications with individuals, families, groups, and communities.

- Demonstrates systems-level critical thinking and communication skills.

- Utilizes systems-level methods to disseminate information.

- Mentors others in presentation and dissemination skills.

- Documents communications so as to promote accountability in practice and to assure compliance with regulatory requirements.

Standard 12. Leadership

The public health nurse demonstrates leadership in the professional practice setting and the profession.

COMPETENCIES

The public health nurse:

- Oversees the nursing care given by others while retaining accountability for the quality of public health nursing care provided.

- Abides by the vision, the associated goals, and the plan to implement and measure progress of an individual, family, community, or population.

- Acts in accordance with organizational goals, including participation in emergency preparedness and response activities.

- Facilitates development of organizational plans to implement programs and policies.

- Participates in teams to assure compliance with organizational policies.

- Mentors colleagues in the acquisition of clinical knowledge, skills, abilities, and judgment.

- Treats colleagues with respect, trust, and dignity.

- Demonstrates a commitment to lifelong learning.

- Demonstrates conflict resolution skills.

- Contributes to promoting a culturally responsive work environment.

- Participates in professional organizations.

- Seeks ways to advance nursing autonomy and accountability.

- Articulates nursing and public health knowledge and skills to the interdisciplinary team, administrators, educators, policy-makers, and appropriate intersectoral partners.

- Participates in efforts to influence healthcare policy to increase access to care, improve quality of care provided, and ensure ethical and equitable provision of care.

ADDITIONAL COMPETENCIES FOR THE ADVANCED
PUBLIC HEALTH NURSE

The advanced public health nurse:

- Influences decision-making bodies to improve the professional practice environment and health outcomes.

- Provides direction to enhance the effectiveness of the interprofessional team.

- Promotes advanced public health nursing and role development by interpreting its role for populations, partners, and others.

- Models expert practice to intersectoral team members, interprofessional colleagues, and others.

- Mentors colleagues for the advancement of nursing practice, the profession, and quality public health services.

Standard 13. Collaboration

The public health nurse collaborates with the population and others in the conduct of nursing practice.

COMPETENCIES

The public health nurse:

- Partners with key individuals, groups, coalitions, and organizations to effect change in public health policies, programs, and services to generate positive outcomes.

- Partners with others in assessing, planning, implementing, and evaluating population-focused policies, programs, and services.

- Communicates with constituencies in the community to gather information and develop partnerships and coalitions to navigate population-focused health concerns.

- Participates in building consensus and resolving conflict in the context of policies, programs, and services.

- Applies group process and negotiation techniques with individuals, families, groups, and communities, as well as with colleagues.

- Adheres to the standards and applicable codes of conduct that govern behavior among peers and colleagues, so as to create a work environment that promotes cooperation, respect, and trust.

- Documents the actions related to policies, programs, and services that indicate collaboration with populations and with others.

- Engages in teamwork and team-building processes.

ADDITIONAL COMPETENCIES FOR THE ADVANCED PUBLIC HEALTH NURSE

The advanced public health nurse:

- Partners as part of alliances and coalitions with local, state, regional, and national organizations to address and sustain public health policies, programs, and services.

- Initiates collaborative efforts across constituencies in the population in order to achieve optimal outcomes.

- Designs education, administrative, research, and public policy programs to promote the health of the populations.

- Leads in establishing, improving, and sustaining collaborative relationships to promote population health.

- Identifies opportunities for collaborative relationships with local, state, regional, and national sources.

- Documents communications, rationales for changes, and collaborative discussions related to public health policies, programs, and services to improve population outcomes.

Standard 14. Professional Practice Evaluation

The public health nurse evaluates her or his own nursing practice in relation to professional practice standards and guidelines, relevant statutes, rules, and regulations.

COMPETENCIES

The public health nurse:

- Implements age-appropriate, population-focused policies, programs, and services in a culturally and ethnically sensitive manner.

- Engages in self-evaluation of practice on a regular basis, identifying areas of strength as well as areas in which professional development would be beneficial.

- Obtains informal feedback regarding her or his practice from community, professional colleagues, peers, and others.

- Participates in peer review as appropriate.

- Takes action to achieve goals identified during the evaluation process.

- Integrates the knowledge of current practice standards, guidelines, statutes, rules, and regulations into her or his work plans.

- Provides the evidence for practice decisions and actions as part of the informal and formal evaluation processes.

- Applies knowledge of current practice standards, guidelines, statutes, certification, and regulation in self-evaluation and peer review.

- Identifies internal and external factors affecting public health nursing practice and services.

- Interacts with peers and colleagues to enhance her or his professional nursing practice or role performance.

- Provides peers with formal or informal constructive feedback regarding their practice or role performance.

- Articulates the benefits of a diverse public health workforce.

- Adapts the delivery of public health nursing care in consideration of changes in the public health system, and the larger social, political, and economic environment.

ADDITIONAL COMPETENCIES FOR THE ADVANCED
PUBLIC HEALTH NURSE

The advanced public health nurse:

- Engages in a formal, systematic process seeking feedback regarding her or his practice from peers, professional colleagues, community and professional organizations, and stakeholders.

- Analyzes her or his practice in relation to advanced certification requirements as appropriate.

Standard 15. Resource Utilization

The public health nurse utilizes appropriate resources to plan and provide nursing and public health services that are safe, effective, and financially responsible.

COMPETENCIES

The public health nurse:

- Assesses the population's available resources to achieve desired health outcomes.

- Identifies the population's needs, potential for harm, complexity, and desired outcomes when considering resource allocation.

- Delegates tasks taking into consideration the concerns of the population, potential for exposure or harm, complexity of the task, and predictability of the outcomes.

- Identifies the evidence when evaluating resources.

- Utilizes community assets and resources to promote health and to deliver care to individuals, families, and groups.

- Advocates for resources, including technology, to enhance nursing practice and for population programs and services.

- Modifies practice when necessary to promote positive interaction among populations, providers, and technology.

- Assists representatives of specific populations and other stakeholders in identifying and securing appropriate and available services to address health-related needs.

- Assists the population to become informed about the options, costs, risks, and benefits of policies, programs, and services.

- Describes the impact of budget constraints on the delivery of public health nursing care to individuals, families, groups, and communities.

- Provides input into budget priorities.

- Provides input into the fiscal and narrative components of proposals for funding from external sources.

ADDITIONAL COMPETENCIES FOR THE ADVANCED
PUBLIC HEALTH NURSE

The advanced public health nurse:

- Utilizes organizational and community resources to formulate inter-sectoral plans for policies, programs, and services.

- Demonstrates fiscal responsibility and integrity in the policy development process.

- Formulates innovative approaches to community and public health concerns that include effective resource utilization and improvement of quality.

- Designs evaluation strategies to demonstrate cost-effectiveness, cost-benefit, and efficiency factors associated with nursing and public health practice and outcomes.

Standard 16. Environmental Health

The public health nurse practices in an environmentally safe, fair, and just manner.

COMPETENCIES

The public health nurse:

- Maintains current knowledge of environmental health concepts, such as implementation of environmental health strategies.

- Promotes a practice environment that reduces environmental health risks for individuals, communities, or populations.

- Assesses the practice environment for factors such as biological, chemical, physical, and psychosocial hazards that threaten health.

- Advocates for the judicious and appropriate use and disposal of products in the home, industry, and community.

- Communicates environmental health risks and exposure reduction strategies to healthcare consumers, families, colleagues, and communities.

- Utilizes scientific evidence and the precautionary principle to determine if a product, practice, or policy is an environmental or human health threat.

- Participates in strategies to promote healthy communities.

- Creates partnerships that promote sustainable environmental health policies and conditions.

- Critically evaluates environmental health issues that are presented by the media.

- Advocates for implementation of environmental principles for nursing practice and public health.

ADDITIONAL COMPETENCIES FOR THE ADVANCED PUBLIC HEALTH NURSE

The advanced public health nurse:

- Analyzes the impact of economic, political, and social influences on the environment and human health exposures.

- Supports nurses in advocating for and implementing environmental principles in nursing practice and public health.

- Designs environmental health programs with community and intersectoral partners and interprofessional experts to assure a healthy and safe environment for all.

Standard 17. Advocacy

The public health nurse advocates for the protection of the health, safety, and rights of the population.

COMPETENCIES

The public health nurse:

- Identifies policy issues relevant to the health of individuals, families, groups, communities, and population.

- Identifies implications of policy options for public health programs and the potential impacts on individuals, communities, and population.

- Integrates advocacy into the implementation of policies, programs, and services for the population.

- Evaluates the effectiveness of advocating for the population when assessing the expected outcomes.

- Demonstrates skill in advocating before providers and stakeholders on behalf of the population.

- Uses conflict resolution skills among populations, providers, and other stakeholders to ensure the safety and guard the best interests of the population and to preserve the professional integrity of the nurse.

- Advocates for equitable access to preventive, health promotion, primary care, and other healthcare services.

ADDITIONAL COMPETENCIES FOR THE ADVANCED PUBLIC HEALTH NURSE

The advanced public health nurse:

- Demonstrates skill in advocating before public representatives and decision-makers on behalf of the populations, programs, and services.

- Designs materials for the advocacy process that are based on the needs of the populations, programs, and services.

Glossary

Advocacy. The act of pleading or arguing in favor of a cause, idea, or policy on someone else's behalf, with a focus on developing the community, system, individual, or family's capacity to plead their own cause or act on their own behalf.

Assessment. The regular and systematic collection, analysis, and dissemination of information on the health of the community or population, including statistics on health status, community health needs, and epidemiological and other studies of health problems.

Assets. The aspects or qualities of a population that can be used to strengthen or enhance population-based initiatives.

Assurance. Making certain that services necessary to achieve agreed-upon goals are provided, by encouraging actions by other entities (private or public), by requiring such action through regulation, or by providing services directly.

Coalition building. The process by which parties (individuals, organizations, or groups) come together to collaborate in working together for a common purpose and to enhance each other's capacity for mutual benefit and common purpose.

Collaboration. Work with another person or group to achieve something.

Community. A collective whole made up of persons in interaction, being and experiencing together, who may or may not share a sense of place or belonging, and who act intentionally for a common purpose. A community is different from the group of people who constitute it and is an interactional whole.

Community-based organizations. Private nonprofit organizations or other types of groups that work within a community for the improvement of some aspect of that community.

Cultural competence. A set of congruent behaviors, attitudes, and policies that come together in a system, agency, or among professionals that enable the system, agency, or professionals to work effectively in cross-cultural situations.

Cultural diversity. The coexistence of different ethnic, gender, racial, and socioeconomic groups.

Determinants of health. Social, economic, and healthcare factors that affect health and well-being independently, and in conjunction with each other, at the population or community level. Comprehensive factors involve relevant social, economic, environmental, behavioral, political, health, and health-care indicators that describe the essential features of a social structure and system and the processes through which change occurs.

Ecological model. A model of health that emphasizes the linkages and relationships among multiple factors (or determinants) affecting health.

Environmental health. Those aspects of human health, including quality of life, that are determined by physical, chemical, biological, social, and psychological processes in the environment. It also refers to the theory and practice of assessing, correcting, controlling, and preventing those factors in the environment that can potentially adversely affect the health of the present and future generations.

Epidemiology. The study of the distribution of determinants and antecedents of health and disease in human populations. The ultimate goal is to identify the underlying causes of a disease and then to apply findings to disease prevention and health promotion.

Evidence. Verifiable knowledge on which to base belief and action.

Evidence-based practice. An approach to public health care practice in which the public health nurse is aware of the evidence in support of his or her clinical practice, and the strength of that evidence.

Health status (of the population). The level of illness or wellness of a population at a designated time.

Interdisciplinary team. A group of individuals who rely on each other's overlapping skills and discipline-based knowledge to achieve synergistic effects whereby outcomes are enhanced and more comprehensive than the simple aggregation of each individual member's efforts.

Intersectoral. Describes working with more than one sector of society to take action on an area of shared interest. Sectors may include government departments such as health, education, environment, and justice; ordinary citizens; nonprofit societies or organizations; and business.

Multisector team. A partnership of community organizations and groups representing a variety of viewpoints and perspectives that impact public health issues.

Outcomes. Long-term objectives that define optimal, measurable future levels of health status; maximum acceptable levels of disease, injury, or dysfunction; or prevalence of risk factors.

Partnership. A relationship in which two or more people or groups operate together as partners. A *partner* is defined as an associate who works with others toward a common goal.

Performance improvement. A process that considers the organizational context, describes desired performance, identifies gaps between desired and actual performance, identifies root causes, selects interventions to close the gaps, and measures changes in performance with the goal of achieving desired results or outcomes.

Policy development. Application of comprehensive public health scientific knowledge for decision-making. Policy development includes a systematic course of action to establish priorities; determine effective strategies and interventions; and use community resources, including regulation and law, to achieve the community's goals.

Population. Those living in a specific geographic area (e.g., a neighborhood, community, city, or county) or those in a particular group (e.g., racial, ethnic, age) who experience a disproportionate burden of poor health outcomes.

Population-focused. An approach to health care that addresses the population level of the ecological model.

Precautionary principle. Professional practice guidance to take precautionary measures against an activity that raises a threat, even if the activity has not yet been scientifically proven to be a threat. The principle includes taking action in the face of uncertainty; shifting burdens of proof to those who create risks; analysis of alternatives to potentially harmful activities; and participatory decision-making methods. The precautionary principle takes the life cycle of products or chemicals into account and adds the proactive step of pre-market analysis of environmental harm.

Social justice. The principle that all persons are entitled to have their basic human needs met, regardless of differences in economic status, class, gender, race, ethnicity, citizenship, religion, age, sexual orientation, disability, or health. This includes the eradication of poverty and illiteracy, the establishment of sound environmental policy, and equality of opportunity for healthy personal and social development.

Stakeholder. A person or organization that has a legitimate interest in what the public health entity does.

Standard. An authoritative statement defined and promoted by a profession by which the quality of practice, service, or education can be evaluated.

Strategic national stockpile. Large quantities of medicines, antidotes, and medical supplies needed to respond to a wide range of scenarios where supplies of critical medical items in any jurisdiction would be rapidly depleted; the stockpile is managed by the Centers for Disease Control and Prevention.

Surveillance. The systematic collection, analysis, interpretation, and dissemination of data to assist in the planning, implementation, and evaluation of public health interventions and programs.

References and Bibliography

Agency for Healthcare Research and Quality (AHRQ), U.S. Preventive Services Task Force. (2010). *Guide to community preventive services*. Washington, DC: Author. Retrieved from http://www.thecommunityguide.org/index.html

American Nurses Association. (1999). *Scope and standards of public health nursing*. Washington, DC: American Nurses Publishing.

American Nurses Association. (2001). *Code of ethics for nurses with interpretive statements*. Washington, DC: American Nurses Publishing.

American Nurses Association. (2007). *ANA principles of environmental health for nursing practice with implementation strategies*. Silver Spring, MD: Nursesbooks.org.

American Nurses Association. (2010). *Nursing: Scope and standards of practice, 2nd ed*. Silver Spring, MD: Nursesbooks.org.

American Public Health Association, Public Health Nursing Section. (2006). *Environmental health principles and recommendations for public health nursing*. Washington, DC: Author.

APRN Joint Dialogue Group. (2008). *Consensus model for APRN regulation: Licensure, accreditation, certification, and education*. Retrieved from https://www.ncsbn.org/Consensus_Model_for_APRN_Regulation_July_2008.pdf

Association of State and Territorial Directors of Nursing (ASTDN). (1999). *Public health nursing: A partner for healthy populations*. Washington, DC: American Nurses Association.

Baur, C. (2010). New directions in research on public health and health literacy. *Journal of Health Communication, 15*(Suppl. 2):42–50. doi:10.1080/10810730.2010.499989

Centers for Disease Control and Prevention (CDC). (2010). *National Public Health Performance Standards Program: 10 essential public health services.* Retrieved from http://www.cdc.gov/nphpsp/essentialservices.html

Council on Linkages (CoL). (2010). *Core competencies for public health professionals.* ("A collaborative activity of the Centers for Disease Control and Prevention, the Health Resources and Services Administration, and the Public Health Foundation.") Retrieved from http://www.phf.org/programs/corecompetencies

Institute of Medicine (IOM). (1988). *The future of public health.* Washington, DC: National Academies Press.

Institute of Medicine. (1996). *Primary care: America's health in a new era.* Washington, DC: National Academies Press.

Institute of Medicine. (2003a). *The future of the public's health in the twenty-first century.* Washington, DC: National Academies Press.

Institute of Medicine. (2003b). *Who will keep the public healthy?* Washington, DC: National Academies Press.

Institute of Medicine. (2004). *Health literacy: A prescription to end confusion.* Washington, DC: National Academies Press.

Institute of Medicine. (2011). *The future of nursing: Leading change, advancing health.* Washington, DC: National Academies Press.

Institute of Medicine. (2012). *Primary care and public health: Exploring integration to improve population health.* Washington, DC: National Academies Press.

Kulbok, P. A., & Ervin, N. E. (2012). Nursing science and public health: Contributions to the discipline of nursing. *Nursing Science Quarterly, 1*(25): 37–43. doi:10.1177/0894318411429034

Kutner, M., Greenberg, E., Jin, Y., and Paulsen, C. (2006). *The health literacy of America's adults: Results from the 2003 National Assessment of Adult Literacy* (NCES 2006–483). Washington, DC: National Center for Education Statistics, U.S. Department of Education.

Levin, P. F., Cary, A. H., Kulbok, P., Leffers, J., Molle, M., & Polivka, B. J. (2008). Graduate education for advanced practice public health nursing: At the crossroads. *Public Health Nursing, 25*(2), 176–193.

Public Health Accreditation Board. (2011). *PHAB standards and measures.* Alexandria, VA: Author.

Public Health Leadership Society. (2002). *Principles of ethical practice of public health, version 2.2.* Retrieved from http://www.phls.org

Quad Council of Public Health Nursing Organizations. (1997). *The tenets of public health nursing.* Unpublished white paper.

Quad Council of Public Health Nursing Organizations. (2011). *Quad council competencies for public health nurses.* Retrieved from http://quadcouncilphn.org/

Quad Council of Public Health Nursing Organizations & American Nurses Association. (1999). *Scope and standards of public health nursing practice.* Washington, DC: American Nurses Publishing.

Raffensberger, C., & Tickner, J. (Eds.). (1999). *Protecting public health and the environment: Implementing the precautionary principle.* Washington, DC: Island Press.

U.S. Census Bureau. (2008). *Press release: An older and more diverse nation by midcentury.* Retrieved from http://www.census.gov/newsroom/releases/archives/population/cb08-123.html

U.S. Department of Health and Human Services. (2000). *Healthy people 2010* (2nd ed.), with *Understanding and improving health and objectives for improving health.* 2 vols. Washington, DC: U.S. Government Printing Office.

U.S. Department of Health and Human Services, Office of Disease Prevention and Health Promotion. (2010) *Healthy people 2020.* Washington, DC: Author. Retrieved from http://www.healthypeople.gov/2020/

U.S. Department of Health and Human Services, Office of the Surgeon General. (2011). *National prevention strategy.* Washington, DC: National Prevention Council. Retrieved from http://www.surgeongeneral.gov/initiatives/prevention/strategy/

World Health Organization. (2012). *Strategic directions for strengthening nursing and midwifery services 2011–2015.* Geneva, Switzerland: Author.

Appendix A

Crosswalk of the Tier 1 Core Competencies for Public Health Nursing and *Public Health Nursing: Scope and Standards of Practice, Second Ed.*

This ANA document, *Public Health Nursing: Scope and Standards of Practice, Second Edition,* delineates competencies for practice: The ANA competencies in this book have been written largely to ensure that public health nursing fits within the domain of an ANA-recognized nursing specialty. *Core Competencies for Public Health Nurses* (CCPHN; Quad Council, 2011; see in-text discussion on pages 16–17) were created to ensure that public health nursing fit in the domain of public health science.

To assure public health nurses that these two sets of competencies are neither in competition with nor burdensome to practice, efforts have been made to align the standards and competencies of this document with the PHN Core Competencies document of the Quad Council.* The "crosswalk" (as represented in the tables on the following pages) correlates the ANA PHN standards and their accompanying competencies with the Tier 1 (basic or generalist level) PHN Core Competencies, organized by the eight practice domains of public health nursing:

- Domain 1. Analytical and Assessment

- Domain 2. Policy Development and Program Planning

- Domain 3. Communication

---

* The Quad Council of Public Health Nursing Organizations (http://quadcouncil-phn.org/) addresses the priorities of and advocates for excellence in public health nursing education, practice, leadership, and research. It is comprised of representatives from these groups:
- Association of Public Health Nurses (APHN)
- Association of Community Health Nurse Educators (ACHNE)
- Public Health Nursing Section of the American Public Health Association (PHN-APHA)
- American Nurses Association (ANA)

- Domain 4. Cultural Competency

- Domain 5. Community Dimensions of Practice

- Domain 6. Basic Public Health Sciences

- Domain 7. Financial Planning and Management

- Domain 8. Leadership and Systems Thinking

The Quad Council adopted for its PHN Core Competencies the structure of the Council on Linkages (2010): eight practice domains spanned by three tiers of practice.

DOMAIN 1. ANALYTIC AND ASSESSMENT

PHN Core Competency	Correlating ANA standard
1. Identifies the determinants of health and illness of individuals and families, using multiple sources of data	Standard 1, Assessment
2. Uses epidemiologic data and the ecological perspective to identify health risks for a population. Identifies individual and family assets and needs, values, and beliefs; resources; and relevant environmental factors.	Standard 1, Assessment
3. Identifies variables that measure health and public health conditions.	Standard 1, Assessment
4. Uses valid and reliable methods and instruments for collecting qualitative and quantitative data from multiple sources. Develops a data collection plan using appropriate technology to collect data to inform the care of individuals, families, and groups.	Standard 1, Assessment
5. Identifies sources of public health data and information. Collects, interprets, and documents data in terms that are understandable to all who were involved in the process, including communities.	Standard 1, Assessment
6. Uses valid and reliable data sources to make comparisons for assessment.	Standard 1, Assessment
7. Identifies gaps and redundancies in data sources in a community assessment through work with individuals, families, and communities.	Standard 6, Evaluation
8. Applies ethical, legal, and policy guidelines and principles in the collection, maintenance, use, and dissemination of data and information.	Standard 1, Assessment
9. Describes the public health nursing applications of quantitative and qualitative data.	Standard 2, Population Diagnosis and Priorities
10. Collects quantitative and qualitative data that can be used in the community health assessment process.	Standard 1, Assessment
Assesses data collected as part of the community assessment process to make inferences about individuals, families, and groups.	Standard 2, Population Diagnosis and Priorities
11. Utilizes information technology to collect, analyze, store, and retrieve data related to nursing care of individuals, families, and groups.	Standard 1, Assessment
12. Practices evidence-based public health nursing to promote the health of individuals and families.	Standard 9, Evidence-Based Practice and Research

DOMAIN 2. POLICY DEVELOPMENT AND PROGRAM PLANNING

PHN Core Competency	Correlating ANA standard
1. Identifies policy issues relevant to the health of individuals, families, and groups. Describes the structure of the public health system and its impacts on individuals, families, and groups within a population.	Standard 17, Advocacy Standard 5E, Regulatory Activities
2. Identifies the implications of policy options for public health programs and the potential impacts on individuals, families, and groups within a population.	Standard 17, Advocacy
3. Identifies outcomes of health policy relevant to PHN practice.	Standard 17, Advocacy
4. Collects information that will inform policy decisions. Describes the legislative policy development process. Identifies outcomes of current health policy relevant to PHN practice.	Standard 5E, Regulatory Activities Standard 17, Advocacy
7.* Describes the structure of the public health system. Identifies public health laws and regulations relevant to PHN practice. Provides public health nursing services in a manner consistent with laws and regulations.	Standard 5E, Regulatory Activities
8. Participates as a team member in developing organizational plans to implement programs and policies.	Standard 12, Leadership
9. Participates in teams to assure compliance with organizational policies.	Standard 12, Leadership
10. Assists in the design of an evaluation plan for an individual-, family-, or community-focused program. Participates as a team member to evaluate programs to individuals, families, and groups for their effectiveness and quality.	Standard 6, Evaluation Standard 6, Evaluation; Standard 10, Quality of Practice
11. Understands methods and practices used to identify and access public health information for individuals, families, and groups.	Standard 11, Communication
12. Understands that quality improvement is important to the practice of public health nursing. Participates in quality improvement teams. Describes various approaches used to improve public health processes and systems. Utilizes quality indicators and core measures to identify and address opportunities for improvement in the care of individuals, families, and groups.	Standard 10, Quality of Practice

(* The discontinuity of the numeration of the Domain 2 competencies from 7 onward is due to the numeration sequence straddling Domains 2 and 3.)

DOMAIN 3. COMMUNICATION

PHN Core Competency	Correlating ANA standard
1. Assesses the health literacy of the individuals, families, and groups served.	Standard 1, Assessment
2. Communicates effectively in writing, orally, and electronically. Communicates in a culturally responsive and relevant manner. Communications are characterized by critical thinking.	Standard 11, Communication
3. Solicits input from individuals, families, and groups when planning and delivering health care.	Standard 4, Planning
4. Utilizes a variety of methods to disseminate public health information to individuals, families, and groups within a population.	Standard 5C, Consultation
5. Demonstrates presentation of targeted health information to multiple audiences at a local level, including to groups, peer professionals, and agency peers.	Standard 14, Professional Practice Evaluation
6. Communicates effectively with individuals, families, and groups and as a member of interprofessional team(s).	Standard 11, Communication
7. Articulates the role of public health nursing to internal and external audiences.	Standard 14, Leadership

DOMAIN 4. CULTURAL COMPETENCY

PHN Core Competency	Correlating ANA standard
1. Utilizes the social and ecological determinants of health to work effectively with diverse individuals, families, and groups.	Standard 1, Assessment
2. Uses concepts, knowledge, and evidence of the social determinants of health in the delivery of services to individuals, families, and groups. Utilizes information technology to understand the impact of the social determinants of health on individuals, families, and groups.	Standard 5, Implementation Standard 6, Evaluation
3. Adapts public health nursing care to individuals, families, and groups based on cultural needs and differences.	Standard 6, Evaluation
4. Explains factors contributing to cultural diversity.	Standard 5B, Health Teaching and Health Promotion
5. Articulates the benefits of a diverse public health workforce.	Standard 14, Professional Practice Evaluation
6. Demonstrates culturally appropriate public health nursing practice with individuals, families, groups, and community members. Contributes to promoting a culturally responsive work environment.	Standard 5B, Health Teaching and Health Promotion Standard 12, Leadership

DOMAIN 5. COMMUNITY DIMENSIONS OF PRACTICE

PHN Core Competency	Correlating ANA standard
1. Utilizes an ecological perspective in health assessment, planning, and interventions with individuals, families, and groups.	Standard 1, Assessment Standard 4, Planning Standard 5, Implementation
2. Identifies research issues at a community level. Functions effectively as a member of a community-based participatory research (CBPR) team.	Standard 9, Evidence-based Practice and Research
3. Identifies community partners for PHN practice with individuals, families, and groups.	Standard 13, Collaboration
4. Collaborates with community partners to promote the health of individuals and families within the population.	Standard 13, Collaboration
5. Partners effectively with key stakeholders and groups in care delivery to individuals, families, and groups.	Standards 13, Collaboration
6. Participates effectively in activities that facilitate community involvement.	Standard 5C, Consultation
7. Describes to individuals, families, and groups the role of government and the private and non-profit sectors in the delivery of community health services.	Standard 5E, Regulatory Activities
8. Utilizes community assets and resources to promote health and deliver care to individuals, families, and groups.	Standard 15, Resource Utilization
9. Seeks input from individuals, families, and groups and incorporates it into the plan of care.	Standard 4, Planning
10. Supports public health policies, programs, and resources. Identifies opportunities for population-focused advocacy for individuals, families, and groups.	Standard 5E, Regulatory Activities Standard 17 Advocacy

DOMAIN 6. PUBLIC HEALTH SCIENCES

PHN Core Competency	Correlating ANA standard
1. Incorporates public health and nursing science in the delivery of care to individuals, families, and groups.	Standard 9, Evidence-Based Practice and Research
2. Describes the historical foundation of public health and public health nursing.	Standard 8, Education
3. Describes how individual-, family-, and group-focused programs contribute to meeting the core public health functions and the 10 essential services.	Standard 8, Education

4. Uses basic descriptive epidemiological methods when conducting a health assessment for individuals, families, and groups.	Standard 1, Assessment
5. Interprets research relevant to public health interventions for individuals, families, and groups.	Standard 9, Evidence-Based Practice and Research
6. Accesses public health and other sources of information using informatics and other information technologies.	Standard 5B, Health Teaching and Health Promotion Standard 6, Evaluation
7. Identifies gaps in research evidence to guide public health nursing practice.	Standard 9, Evidence-Based Practice and Research
8. Complies with the requirements of patient confidentiality and human subject protection.	Standard 7, Ethics
9. Participates in research at the community level to build the scientific base of public health nursing.	Standard 9, Evidence-Based Practice and Research

DOMAIN 7. FINANCIAL PLANNING AND MANAGEMENT

PHN Core Competency	Correlating ANA standard
1. Describes the interrelationships among local, state, tribal, and federal public health and healthcare systems.	Standard 13, Collaboration
2. Describes the structure, function, and jurisdictional authority of the organizational units within federal, state, tribal, and local public health agencies.	Standard 5E, Regulatory Activities
3. Adheres to the organization's policies and procedures, including emergency preparedness and response.	Standard 12, Leadership
4. Provides data for inclusion in a programmatic budget.	Standard 15, Resource Utilization
5. Describes the impact of budget constraints on the delivery of public health nursing care to individuals, families, and groups. Contributes to the evaluation plan for a program targeting individuals, families, and/or groups.	Standard 15, Resource Utilization Standard 6, Evaluation
6. Adapts the delivery of public health nursing care to individuals, families, and groups based on reported evaluation results.	Standard 6, Evaluation
7. Provides input into the fiscal and narrative components of proposals for funding from external sources.	Standard 15, Resource Utilization
8. Applies basic human relations and conflict management skills in interactions with peers and other healthcare team members.	Standard 12, Leadership

9. Utilizes public health informatics skills relative to the public health nursing care of individuals, families, and groups.	Standard 8, Education
10. Provides input into contracts and other agreements for the provision of services.	Standard 13, Collaboration
11. Delivers public health nursing care within budgetary guidelines.	Standard 15, Resource Utilization

DOMAIN 8. LEADERSHIP AND SYSTEMS THINKING

PHN Core Competency	Correlating ANA standard
1. Incorporates ethical standards of practice as the basis of all interactions with organizations, communities, and individuals. Incorporates ethical standards into all aspects of PHN practice.	Standard 7, Ethics
2. Applies systems theory to PHN practice with individuals, families, and groups.	Standard 9, Evidence-Based Practice and Research
3. Participates with stakeholders to identify vision, values, and principles for community action.	Standard 12, Leadership
4. Identifies internal and external factors affecting PHN practice and services.	Standard 14, Professional Practice Evaluation
5. Uses individual, team, and organizational learning opportunities for personal and professional development as a public health nurse.	Standard 8, Education
6. Acts as a mentor, coach, or peer advisor/reviewer for public health nursing staff. Maintains personal commitment to lifelong learning and professional development.	Standard 12, Leadership Standard 8, Education
7. Participates in quality initiatives that identify opportunities for improvement. Provides data to measure, report, and improve organizational performance.	Standard 10, Quality of Practice
8. Adapts the delivery of public health nursing care in consideration of changes in the public health system, and the larger social, political, and economic environment. Maintains knowledge of current public health laws and policies relevant to public health nursing practice.	Standard 14, Professional Practice Evaluation Standard 5E, Regulatory Activities

Appendix B.

Public Health Nursing: Scope and Standards of Practice (2007)

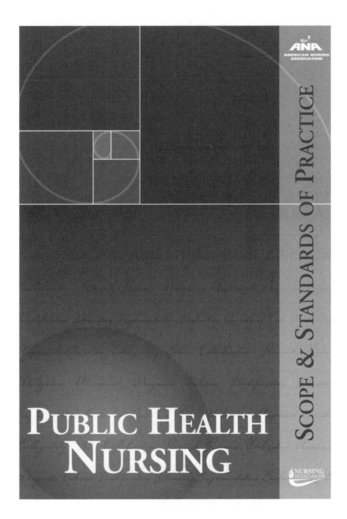

The content in this appendix is not current and is of historical significance only.

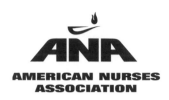

**AMERICAN NURSES
ASSOCIATION**

PUBLIC HEALTH NURSING:
SCOPE AND STANDARDS
OF PRACTICE

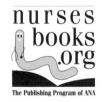

AMERICAN NURSES ASSOCIATION
SILVER SPRING, MARYLAND
2007

The content in this appendix is not current and is of historical significance only.

Library of Congress Cataloging-in-Publication data

Public health nursing : scope and standards of practice /American Nurses Association.
   p. ; cm.
   Includes bibliographical references and index.
   ISBN-13: 978-1-55810-246-0 (pbk.)
   ISBN-10: 1-55810-246-9 (pbk.)
     1. Public health nursing.   2. Community health nursing.   3. Public health
nursing—Practice.   4. Public health nursing—Study and teaching.   I. American
Nurses Association.
   [DNLM: 1. Public Health Nursing—standards—Guideline.   2. Community Health
Nursing—Guideline.   3. Nurse's Role—Guideline. WY 108 P9768 2007]

RT97.P8376 2007
   610.73'4—dc22   2006101337

The American Nurses Association (ANA) is a national professional association. This ANA publication— *Public Health Nursing: Scope and Standards of Practice*—reflects the thinking of the nursing profession on various issues and should be reviewed in conjunction with state board of nursing policies and practices. State law, rules, and regulations govern the practice of nursing, while *Public Health Nursing: Scope and Standards of Practice* guides nurses in the application of their professional skills and responsibilities.

Published by Nursesbooks.org
The Publishing Program of ANA

American Nurses Association
8515 Georgia Avenue, Suite 400
Silver Spring, MD 20910-3492
1-800-274-4ANA
http://www.nursesbooks.org/

ANA is the only full-service professional organization representing the nation's 2.7 million Registered Nurses through its 54 constituent member associations. ANA advances the nursing profession by fostering high standards of nursing practice, promoting the economic and general welfare of nurses in the workplace, projecting a positive and realistic view of nursing, and lobbying the Congress and regulatory agencies on healthcare issues affecting nurses and the public.

Page design: Scott Bell, Arlington, VA ~ *Cover design*: Freedom by Design, Alexandria, VA ~ *Composition*: House of Equations, Inc., Arden, NC ~ *Proofreading*: Lisa Munsat Anthony, Chapel Hill, NC ~ *Editing & Indexing*: Steven A. Jent, Denton, TX ~ *Printing*: McArdle Printing, Upper Marlboro, MD

First printing December 2006.

ISBN-13: 978-1-55810-246-0   ISBN-10: 1-55810-236-9   SAN: 851-3481
05SSPH   3M   12/06

The content in this appendix is not current and is of historical significance only.

ACKNOWLEDGMENTS

Work Group Members

Joy F. Reed, EdD, RN, Chairperson
Betty Bekemeier, MSN, MPH, RN
Kaye Bender, RN, PhD, FAAN
M. Beth Benedict, DrPH, JD, RN
Ellen L. Bridge, BS, MT, RN
Stephanie Chalupka, EdD, APRN, BC, FAAOHN
Mary Pat Couig, MPH, RN, FAAN
Philip A. Greiner, DNSc, RN
Glenda Kelly, MSN, RN
Joan Kub, PhD, APRN, BC
Pamela A. Kulbok, DNSc, APRN, BC
Deborah S. Martz, BSN, RN

ANA Staff

Carol J. Bickford, PhD, RN, BC—Content editor
Yvonne Daley Humes, MSA—Project coordinator
Matthew Seiler, RN, Esq.—Legal counsel

Winifred Carson-Smith, JD—Legal consultant

The content in this appendix is not current and is of historical significance only.

CONTENTS

The content in this appendix is not current and is of historical significance only.

The content in this appendix is not current and is of historical significance only.

PREFACE

Public Health Nursing: Scope and Standards of Practice outlines the expectations of the professional role within which all public health registered nurses should practice. This scope statement and these updated standards of public health nursing practice are meant to guide, define, and direct public health professional nursing practice in all settings.

The American Nurses Association (ANA) has actively engaged in scope of practice and standards development initiatives since the late 1960s. ANA published the first *Standards of Nursing Practice* for the nursing profession in 1973. The standards were generic in nature and focused on the basic nursing process—a critical thinking model applicable to all registered nurses—composed of assessment, diagnosis, outcomes identification, planning, implementation, and evaluation. Over the years, various revisions have ensued, the most recent being *Nursing: Scope and Standards of Practice* (ANA, 2004). Specialty nursing organizations have affirmed this work by using the template language of the standards when developing scope of practice statements and standards of practice for registered nurses engaged in specialty practice.

The Quad Council of Public Health Nursing Organizations, which represents nurses involved in population-focused and community-oriented nursing practice, collaborated with ANA over several years to create *Scope and Standards of Public Health Nursing Practice* (Quad Council & ANA, 1999). This effort was intended to help meet the growing demand for healthcare professionals dedicated to health promotion and protection services for individuals and populations. Since that time, significant national and global events, such as the HIV/AIDs epidemic, natural disasters, and terrorist attacks within the United States, have intensified individual and population concerns.

As part of its regular scope and standards of nursing practice development, review, and maintenance processes, the ANA convened a volunteer work group of public health and community health nursing stakeholders in 2004 to review and revise the 1999 *Scope and Standards of Public Health Nursing Practice* to best reflect contemporary public health nursing practice and set a framework for future practice. ANA specifically charged this work group to review and incorporate relevant content from the 1986 *Standards of Community Health Nursing*. After

The content in this appendix is not current and is of historical significance only.

careful review and consideration, the work group determined that the 2006 *Public Health Nursing: Scope and Standards of Practice* would fully incorporate and replace that 1986 document. The work group also made a conscious decision to use *Advanced Practice Public Health Nurse* to denote the second level of practice (i.e., clinical nurse specialist). This is consistent with and reinforces the ANA position that the clinical nurse specialist is one of the four advanced practice roles in nursing.

The work group:

- analyzed numerous reports and publications of the Institute of Medicine (IOM), the American Public Health Association (APHA), and other organizations as part of an environmental assessment,

- sought comment on a draft model and standards from attendees at a special forum at the 2004 fall APHA meeting,

- notified ANA's constituent member associations, specialty nursing organizations, public health organizations, and other stakeholders that input was requested on the draft document,

- posted the draft document on ANA's www.NursingWorld.org web site for public review and comment by interested nurses and others,

- considered all public suggestions posted during the comment period, and

- finalized the draft document for submission to the ANA review and publication process.

The ANA review included evaluation by the Committee on Nursing Practice Standards and Guidelines of ANA's Congress on Nursing Practice and Economics for compliance with established criteria. The Congress on Nursing Practice and Economics then completed another level of review, culminating in the approval of the specialty scope of practice statement and acknowledgment of the specialty nursing standards of practice.

The goal of public health nursing is to improve the health and well-being of all individuals, families, communities, and populations through the significant and visible contributions of registered nurses utilizing standards-based practice. This goal will be achieved when the contents of this document are consistently applied to practice, education, and research. For example, the scope and standards for public health nurs-

The content in this appendix is not current and is of historical significance only.

ing may be used as the basis for developing public health nursing job descriptions and performance evaluations. In the population-focused nursing education domain, the scope and standards can guide curriculum development. Finally, the rich content of the public health nursing scope and standards of practice can provide direction for expanding the focus of the public health nursing research agenda.

The content in this appendix is not current and is of historical significance only.

PUBLIC HEALTH NURSING: SCOPE OF PRACTICE

Context for Twenty-first Century Public Health Nursing Practice

For over a century, public health nursing has significantly contributed to population-focused health through effective partnerships. Beginning in the early part of the twentieth century, Lillian Wald, Lavinia Dock, and their nursing colleagues at the Henry Street Settlement House in New York's Lower East Side applied spirited innovation to organize themselves and others, working in and with communities to heal, partner, mobilize, support, and bring about change in the disadvantaged populations in which they lived and worked. Such partnerships continue today as public health nurses work with communities and populations to identify specific public health assets and needs, addressing those issues at multiple levels, and using the political process to assure the health of communities.

Several reports and events have influenced how public health nurses conceptualize and define the practice of public health nursing for the twenty-first century. The Institute of Medicine's report, *The Future of the Public's Health in the Twenty-first Century* (2003a), builds upon a previous IOM report, *The Future of Public Health* (1988), and contains specific recommendations for strengthening the relationships among the vital sectors charged with protecting the public's health. These sectors include the governmental public health infrastructure, communities (including schools, elected officials, and community and faith-based organizations), healthcare delivery systems, employers and businesses, the media, academia, and the research community.

An ecological approach, proposed by the IOM's 2003 report, is the basis for understanding health in populations. This approach recognizes multiple determinants of health that are critical not only for understanding the concept of health, but also for assuring conditions in which populations may achieve good health. This ecological approach is also based on the assumption that health is influenced at several levels within the ecological framework, such as individuals, families, communities, organizations, and social systems. An ecological approach to public health nursing practice is based on population-focused services and programs, advocacy, research, and education. See Appendix A for a

The content in this appendix is not current and is of historical significance only.

comparison of selected well-known public health nursing intervention models and the multiple determinants of population health using this ecological approach.

Nursing comprises the largest single workforce in the health system. Therefore, nurses have significant opportunities to create an environment that ensures good health. This is especially true in public health nursing practice with its focus on health promotion, disease prevention, and improved health status through nursing care and collaboration with communities. These services and programs often alter the interaction of the determinants of health to produce conditions in which people may attain and maintain health. Recommendations from *The Future of the Public's Health in the Twenty-first Century* (IOM, 2003a) provide direction for defining and creating new approaches in public health nursing practice, education, and research that utilize the ecological model to alter the social determinants of health.

A companion IOM study, *Who Will Keep the Public Healthy?* (2003b), also builds on an ecological approach and considers factors likely to influence public health in the twenty-first century, such as globalization, technological and scientific advances, and demographic shifts in the United States. This IOM report explores issues and lists recommendations regarding further development of the public health workforce. A public health professional is defined in this report as a person educated in public health or a related discipline who is engaged in improving health through a focus on populations.

The report delineates eight new content domains for public health professionals: informatics, genomics, communication, cultural competence, community-based participatory research, policy and law, global health, and ethics. These content areas are proposed to assist the present and future public health workforce to meet the emerging needs of new global public health issues and advances in science and policy. Both IOM reports emphasize the vision of the national health objectives for healthy people in healthy communities as described in *Healthy People 2010* (HHS, 2000; http://www.healthypeople.gov/Publications/).

The development of public health competencies by the Council on Linkages Between Academia and Public Health Practice (2001) is another landmark effort with potential influence on the public health nursing specialty. These competencies provide direction for the education, practice, and future research of public health professionals.

The content in this appendix is not current and is of historical significance only.

The Quad Council of Public Health Nursing Organizations, an alliance of the Association of Community Health Nursing Educators (ACHNE), the American Nurses Association 's (ANA) Congress on Nursing Practice and Economics, the American Public Health Association Public Health Nursing Section, and the Association of State and Territorial Directors of Nursing (ASTDN), developed public health nursing specific competencies (Quad Council of Public Health Nursing Organizations, 2004), using the Council on Linkages competencies as a framework (Council on Linkages Between Academia and Practice, 2001). These public health nursing competencies were designed to be used with other documents, such as *The Definition and Role of Public Health Nursing* (APHA PHN Section, 1996) and the 1999 edition of the *Scope and Standards of Public Health Nursing Practice* (Quad Council & ANA, 1999). The public health nursing competencies called attention to the population-focused nature of public health nursing practice and emphasized how public health nursing is unique in its approach to health improvement at the individual, family, community, and population levels.

Another set of documents to be considered in guiding the work of public health nursing for the twenty-first century is the *National Public Health Performance Standards* (CDC, 2001). These standards define optimal performance at the state, local, and federal levels of public health and are designed to guide self-assessment and quality improvement activities for the operation of public health systems well into the future. For the NPHPS assessment, the public health system is defined in its broadest context, similar to the ecological model used in the 2003 IOM report, and considers all partners with a role in improving and protecting the public's health.

Public health nursing practice in the United States is becoming increasingly complex. Societal and political changes have contributed to this complexity. Threats to the health of populations include a re-emergence of communicable diseases, increasing incidence of drug-resistant organisms, overall concern about the structure of the healthcare system, environmental hazards, and the challenges imposed by the presence of modern public health epidemics such as obesity- and tobacco-related deaths.

Global and emerging crises have increased the vulnerability of populations to multiple health threats. These threats have dramatically redirected attention toward public health preparedness with its new priorities and activities, such as syndromic surveillance, mass casualty planning, and the handling of biological and chemical agents as evidentiary material as well as for removal of a public health hazard. Postal workers, law enforcement personnel, and communications experts are among the new groups that have emerged as partners with public health nurses (IOM, 1995).

Public health nurses exhibit leadership in many of these emerging priority public health initiatives. These roles provide opportunities for public health nurses to determine the evidence by which new public health system changes are implemented and evaluated, and then to develop operational systems that can be effectively deployed for any emerging public health threat. Similarly, public health nurses are also increasingly identified as leaders in public health system reform.

During the twenty-first century there is likely to be an even greater emphasis on population-focused services in public health demanding new knowledge and skills of public health nurses. The practice of public health nurses of this century will be guided not only by sound application of evidence-based intervention models, but also by these sources:

- Current scope and standards of practice for public health nursing

- Core functions of public health (IOM, 1988)

- Ten Essential Public Health Services (http://www.cdc.gov/od/ocphp/nphpsp/EssentialPHServices.htm)

- *Definition and Role of Public Health Nursing* (APHA, 1996)

- Quad Council Public Health Nursing Competencies (2004)

- *Healthy People 2010,* (HHS, 2000)

- *National Public Health Performance Standards* (CDC, 2001)

- *Essentials of Baccalaureate Nursing Education for Entry Level Community Health Nursing Practice* (ACHNE, 2000)

- *Essentials of Master's Level Nursing Education for Advanced Community/Public Health Nursing Practice* (ACHNE, 2003)

- An ecological approach model similar to that described in *The Future of the Public's Health in the Twenty-first Century* (IOM, 2003a)

The content in this appendix is not current and is of historical significance only.

Definition of Public Health Nursing

Public health nursing is the practice of promoting and protecting the health of populations using knowledge from nursing, social, and public health sciences (American Public Health Association, Public Health Nursing Section, 1996). The practice is population-focused with the goals of promoting health and preventing disease and disability for all people through the creation of conditions in which people can be healthy.

Although practicing in a variety of public and private organizations, all public health nurses focus on one or more populations. A population may be defined as those living in a specific geographic area (e.g., a neighborhood, community, city or county) or those in a particular group (e.g., racial, ethnic, age, disease) who experience a disproportionate burden of poor health outcomes.

Population-based public health nursing practice focuses on entire populations that possess similar health concerns or characteristics. This includes everyone in a population who is actually or potentially affected by a health concern or shares a specific characteristic. Population-based public health nursing interventions are not limited to those who seek service, are poor, or otherwise vulnerable. Public health nursing services and programs may be directed toward entire populations within a community, the systems that affect the health of those populations, or the individuals and families within those populations. The public health nurse partners with communities and populations to reduce health risks and to promote, maintain, and restore health, advocating for system-level changes to improve health.

Public health nurses must understand and apply concepts from various disciplines, including community organization and development, coordination of care, health education and maintenance, and environmental health, in addition to nursing and public health sciences. Public health nurses practice in partnership with the population and numerous other groups, including:

- members of the public health team such as epidemiologists, social workers, nutritionists, environmental health workers, and health educators;
- local, state, and federal public health organizations;
- healthcare providers;

The content in this appendix is not current and is of historical significance only.

- community organizations and coalitions;

- community service agencies such as schools, law enforcement, and emergency response;

- faith-based organizations;

- businesses and industries; and

- academic and research institutions.

Public health nurses work to improve health at the individual, family, community, and population levels through the core functions of assessment, assurance, and policy development (IOM, 1988). The core functions are applied in a systematic and comprehensive manner.

Assessment includes a review of the concerns, strengths, and expectations of the population and is guided by epidemiological methods and the nursing process.

Assurance is accomplished through regulation, advocating for other healthcare professionals to provide needed services, coordinating community services, or, at times, direct provision of services. Assurance strategies take into account the availability, acceptability, accessibility, and quality and effectiveness of services. Public health nurses focus on assurance activities and initiatives that provide appropriate service delivery to achieve targeted outcomes and that monitor health service access, utilization, and appropriateness for the community, including underserved and target populations. In addition, assurance functions include participation in developing systems and programs to promote positive health outcomes for the community, working to implement continuous quality improvement for healthcare systems in the community, and providing expert public health nurse consultation to groups and organizations in the community.

The necessary policies are developed according to the results of the assessment, the priorities set by the population, and consideration of subpopulations and communities at greatest risk, as well as the evidence on effectiveness of various activities or strategies.

Public health nurses are proactive with respect to social and healthcare trends, changing concerns, and policy and legislative activities. They function as advocates for the populations they serve. Such advocacy for public health and social policies promotes a healthy environment, cre-

The content in this appendix is not current and is of historical significance only.

ates conditions that improve and enhance the health of populations, and is a key part of public health nursing roles.

Public health nurses engage in research that enhances public health nursing practice and documents the outcomes of specific activities and strategies. They have an obligation to actively enhance the science and evidence base for professional practice. A clear and well-documented evidence base for public health nursing practice permits the use of the most efficient, effective, and cost-beneficial strategies in promoting the public's health.

When public health nurses partner with individuals, the focus becomes the promotion of knowledge, attitudes, beliefs, practices, and behaviors that support and enhance health, with the ultimate goal of improving the overall health of the population. Similarly, activities with families and communities aim at promoting family and community norms, attitudes, awareness, and behaviors that improve the family's or community's overall health. Activities with populations address organizations, policies, and laws, and include key stakeholders that affect the environment in which people reside and create conditions which allow or promote health for all.

Distinguishing Public Health Nursing from Other Nursing Specialties

Public health nurses enter the specialty from diverse educational and practice backgrounds. While public health nursing practice is traditionally associated with nurses employed by governmental agencies, such as state, local, and tribal health departments, the work also occurs in settings such as community- or faith-based organizations, health maintenance organizations, and community health centers. For purposes of this document, the definition of a public health professional cited in *Who Will Keep the Public Healthy?* describes the work of public health nurses, regardless of their employment setting: "A public health professional is a person educated in public health or a related discipline who is employed to improve health through a population focus" (IOM, 2003b).

Grounded in both the nursing and the public health sciences, public health nursing is distinguished from other nursing specialties by its adherence to *all* of the following eight principles:

The content in this appendix is not current and is of historical significance only.

- *The client or* unit of care *is the population.* While a public health nurse may engage in activities with individuals, families, or groups, the dominant responsibility is to the population as a whole.

- *The primary obligation is to achieve the greatest good for the greatest number of people or the population as a whole.* Public health nurses recognize that it may not be possible to meet individual needs if those needs conflict with priority health goals that benefit the whole population.

- *The processes used by public health nurses include working with the client as an equal partner.* The public health nurse's actions must reflect awareness of the need for comprehensive health planning in partnership with communities and populations and include the perspectives, priorities, and values of the population in interpreting the data, making policy and program decisions, and selecting appropriate strategies for action.

- *Primary prevention is the priority in selecting appropriate activities.* Primary prevention includes health promotion and health protection strategies.

- *Public health nursing focuses on strategies that create healthy environmental, social, and economic conditions in which populations may thrive.* Public health nursing interventions include education, community development, social engineering, policy development, and enforcement. Such interventions emerge from work with the population and result in laws and rules, policies, and budget priorities. Advocating for and teaching advocacy skills to others to create healthy conditions is an essential part of public health nursing practice.

- *A public health nurse is obligated to actively identify and reach out to all who might benefit from a specific activity or service.* Because risk factors are not randomly distributed, specific subpopulations may be more vulnerable to disease or disability or may have more difficulty in accessing or using services, thus requiring special outreach. Public health nurses focus on the whole population and not just those who present for services.

- *Optimal use of available resources to assure the best overall improvement in the health of the population is a key element of the practice.* Public health nurses must be involved in organizing and coordinat-

The content in this appendix is not current and is of historical significance only.

ing the actions of others in response to health issues. In addition, they must use and provide information to other decision-makers regarding the scientific evidence related to outcomes of specific actions, programs, or policies, as well as the cost-effectiveness of potential strategies. Public health nurses must also strive to create the evidence where it is lacking.

- *Collaboration with a variety of other professions, populations, organizations, and other stakeholder groups is the most effective way to promote and protect the health of the people.* Creating the conditions in which people can be healthy is an extremely complex, resource-intensive process. Public health nurses join with appropriate experts from a variety of fields and professions, as well as community members, in efforts to improve population health. This includes public health nurses' recognition of the importance of legislative action and involvement in other means by which health and social policies are set at all levels. This collaboration may occur within the healthcare system or the government; it promotes adoption or revision of such policies.

Ethical Responsibilities

Public health nurses are bound by the ethical provisions for all nurses made explicit in *Code of Ethics for Nurses with Interpretive Statements* (ANA, 2001), *Principles of Ethical Practice of Public Health* (Public Health Leadership Society, 2002), and *Environmental Health Principles and Recommendations for Public Health Nursing* (APHA, 2006). In working with populations, public health nurses must acknowledge the right of the population to have access to the necessary information and opportunities for dialogue in order to make informed decisions without coercion.

Advances in scientific, medical, and healthcare technologies create ethical and legal questions that must be addressed while respecting the diverse values, beliefs, and cultures present in the population served. The need to receive or share information concerning an individual's health in order to protect the health of the public creates a unique set of ethical issues for public health nurses. Likewise, the promise of genomics for contributing to the understanding of and ability to prevent morbidity and mortality must be tempered by the possibility of using such information to further disenfranchise and limit access to care for certain populations.

The content in this appendix is not current and is of historical significance only.

The purpose of public health nursing science is to enhance the health of populations. Public health nurses must recognize and establish their professional practice in accordance with the populations' rights and with a particular concern for social justice. This includes using the Precautionary Principle to guide practice and engage in preventive actions in the face of uncertainty, exploring a wide range of alternatives to potentially harmful actions, and promoting increased public participation in decision-making (Tickner, 2002; Tickner & Raffensberger, 1998). In addition, when making decisions that have an impact on health, public health nurses are obligated to assure that ethical issues are addressed as part of the decision-making process. Public health nurses should also be represented on ethics bodies that make decisions that affect the rights of the population and public health nurses.

Education

The baccalaureate degree in nursing is the educational credential for entry into public health nursing practice. Master's level education is assumed for the nurse specialist level with specific expertise in population-focused care. This educational preparation best prepares public health nurses to function in the specialty role. Associate degree and diploma-prepared registered nurses and licensed practical nurses may appropriately practice in community settings where care is directed toward the health or illness of individuals or families, rather than populations.

In the accompanying standards of practice, the term *advanced practice public health nurse* is used to describe the additional expectations of master's-prepared public health nurses who function as clinical nurse specialists or nurse practitioners in population-focused care (ANA, 2003, 2004a). This advanced practice registered nurse must meet all of the educational and practice criteria required for both generalist and specialist public health nursing practice. Public health nurses who function in nurse administrator roles should additionally use *Scope and Standards for Nurse Administrators* (ANA, 2004b).

Many public health nursing roles require knowledge, skills, and abilities at the doctoral level. Multiple venues for pursuing doctoral level education exist, and program selection may depend on the role the public health nurse holds or wishes to hold (e.g., clinical practice or research, interdisciplinary public health, informatics, epidemiology, ethics).

The content in this appendix is not current and is of historical significance only.

The individual public health nurse pursuing a doctorate needs to assure that the population focus is a central component of the selected course of study.

All public health nurses are expected to be lifelong learners. This means they actively engage in a process of self-assessment to review their current knowledge, skills, and abilities to identify areas for further development. Such professional development may include enrollment in a formal academic program or participation in continuing education studies. Specialty certification in public health nursing is available from the American Nurses Credentialing Center (ANCC) for the public health/community health clinical nurse specialist.

Summary

Public health nursing has historically responded to the needs of populations through effective partnerships. Promoting and protecting population health in the twenty-first century requires that public health nurses have an understanding of the multiple determinants of health. This ecological approach to health is critical as public health nurses not only respond to the health concerns of individuals and communities, but are proactive in the development and implementation of programs and policies to enhance the health of populations. Public health nursing emphasizes the core functions and essential services of public health. The role of the public health nurse is distinguished from other nursing specialties by its emphasis on population-focused services with goals of promoting health and preventing disease and disability, as well as improving quality of life. Public health nurses work to create environmental conditions to assure health through collaboration with a variety of other professions, organizations, and communities. In the context of an evolving healthcare system for the twenty-first century, public health nurses are valued members of the public health workforce; they have the knowledge and skills to deal with the threats, barriers, and factors that influence the health of populations.

The content in this appendix is not current and is of historical significance only.

STANDARDS OF PUBLIC HEALTH NURSING PRACTICE

The Standards of Public Health Nursing Practice and the associated measurement criteria are adapted from and reflect the intent of the template language of the Standards of Practice and Standards of Professional Performance presented in *Nursing: Scope and Standards of Practice* (ANA, 2004a).

Standards of Practice

The six Standards of Practice describe a competent level of public health nursing care as demonstrated by the critical thinking model known as the nursing process. The nursing process includes the components of assessment, diagnosis, outcomes identification, planning, implementation, and evaluation. The nursing process encompasses all significant actions taken by registered nurses and forms the foundation of the nurse's decision-making.

Standards of Professional Performance

Taken together the ten Standards of Professional Performance describe competency in the professional role. The standards address a competency level, including activities related to quality of practice, education, professional practice evaluation, collegiality, collaboration, ethics, research, resource utilization, and leadership. The advocacy standard addresses the unique responsibility of all public health nurses to serve as spokespersons for those who cannot address their own healthcare concerns.

Measurement Criteria

Measurement criteria are key indicators of competent practice for each standard. For a standard to be met, all the listed measurement criteria must be met.

Standards should remain stable over time, as they reflect the philosophical values of the profession. Measurement criteria, however, can be

The content in this appendix is not current and is of historical significance only.

revised more frequently to incorporate advancements in scientific knowledge and expectations for nursing practice. Additional measurement criteria that are applicable only to advanced practice registered nurses are included for select standards of practice and professional performance.

Words such as *appropriate* and *possible* are sometimes used because a document like this one cannot account for all situations that the public health nurse may encounter in practice. The registered nurse will need to exercise judgment based on education and experience in determining what is appropriate or possible for a population or situation. Further direction may be available from documents such as guidelines for practice or agency standards, policies, procedures, and protocols.

The content in this appendix is not current and is of historical significance only.

STANDARDS OF PUBLIC HEALTH NURSING PRACTICE
STANDARDS OF PRACTICE

STANDARD 1. ASSESSMENT
The public health nurse collects comprehensive data pertinent to the health status of populations.

Measurement Criteria:

The public health nurse:

- Collects multi-source data related to the health of the public at large or of a specific population.

- Uses models and principles of epidemiology, demography, and biometry, as well as social, behavioral, and physical sciences to structure data collection.

- Sets assessment priorities based on urgency of need or risk in geographic areas or in populations.

- Conducts an assessment based on criteria that aim to capture the population assets and needs, values and beliefs, resources, and relevant environmental factors.

- Analyzes data using problem-solving techniques and models from nursing, public health, and other disciplines.

- Interprets data to identify trends and deviations from expected health patterns in the population.

- Documents assessment data in terms that are understandable to all involved in the process.

- Applies ethical, legal, and privacy guidelines and policies to the collection, maintenance, use, and dissemination of data and information.

Additional Measurement Criteria for the Advanced Practice Public Health Nurse:

The advanced practice public health nurse:

- Gathers data from multiple, interdisciplinary sources using appropriate methods to augment or verify population-focused data.

Continued ▶

The content in this appendix is not current and is of historical significance only.

- Partners with populations, health professionals, and other stakeholders to attach meaning to collected data.

- Synthesizes complex, multi-source data gathered through the assessment process.

- Consults with the public health nurse, the population, the interdisciplinary team, and other stakeholders in the design, management, and evaluation of the data system that focuses on population assets, needs, and concerns.

The content in this appendix is not current and is of historical significance only.

STANDARD 2. POPULATION DIAGNOSIS AND PRIORITIES
The public health nurse analyzes the assessment data to determine the population diagnoses and priorities.

Measurement Criteria:

The public health nurse:

- Derives the population diagnoses and priorities based on assessment data such as:

  - input from the population,

  - data related to access and use of health services,

  - factors contributing to health promotion and disease prevention,

  - existing or potential harmful exposures, and

  - basic nursing and public health-related sciences.

- Validates the diagnoses or concerns with the population; local, state, and federal public health agencies and organizations; and available health data and statistics as applicable.

- Documents diagnoses or concerns in a manner that facilitates population involvement in the determination of the plan and its expected outcomes.

Additional Measurement Criteria for the Advanced Practice Public Health Nurse:

The advanced practice public health nurse:

- Organizes complex data and information obtained during socio-cultural, demographic, health status and health risk, geographic, environmental, and other nursing and public health diagnostic processes to identify population health assets, needs, and risks.

- Systematically analyzes relevant population data, scientific principles, and events in the environment in formulating differential diagnoses and in setting priorities.

The content in this appendix is not current and is of historical significance only.

STANDARD 3. OUTCOMES IDENTIFICATION
The public health nurse identifies expected outcomes for a plan that is based on population diagnoses and priorities.

Measurement Criteria:

The public health nurse:

- Involves the population and other professionals, organizations, and stakeholders in formulating expected outcomes.

- Derives culturally relevant expected outcomes from the diagnoses.

- Considers population values and beliefs, health literacy, risks, benefits, costs, current social policies, current scientific evidence, and expertise when formulating priorities and expected outcomes.

- Incorporates knowledge of environmental factors and events, available resources, time estimates, and ethical, legal, and privacy considerations in defining expected outcomes.

- Develops outcomes that provide continuity in meeting population needs and concerns and enhancing assets.

- Modifies expected outcomes based on changes in population needs or concerns and the availability of resources.

- Documents expected outcomes as measurable objectives using language that is understandable to all involved entities.

- Applies nursing and public health competencies when measuring effective practice in a community or a population.

Additional measurement criteria for the advanced practice public health nurse:

The advanced practice public health nurse:

- Assures that professional partners are involved in identifying expected outcomes that incorporate scientific evidence and are achievable through implementation of evidence-based practices.

- Assures that measurable outcomes include such factors as cost-effectiveness, satisfaction of stakeholders, the population, and organization, continuity and consistency of services, and resolution of health concerns.

The content in this appendix is not current and is of historical significance only.

STANDARD 4. PLANNING

The public health nurse develops a plan that reflects best practices by identifying strategies, action plans, and alternatives to attain expected outcomes.

Measurement Criteria:

The public health nurse:

- Assists with the development of population-focused plans for health-related services or programs based on an assessment and prioritization of health assets, needs, risks, and concerns.

- Incorporates evidence-based approaches for promotion, improvement, and restoration of health; prevention of illness, injury, or disease; and emergency preparedness and response that address the identified assets, needs, and concerns.

- Provides for continuity within and across programs and services.

- Establishes plans that reflect cultural competence, educational and learning principles, and priorities that address the population needs.

- Ensures participation of the identified population, health professionals, coalitions, organizations, and other stakeholders in determining roles within the planning processes.

- Applies current standards, statutes, regulations, and policies in the planning process.

- Integrates current and emerging trends and research in nursing and public health-related fields in the planning process.

- Considers the economic impacts of the plan on the population and organizations.

- Documents the plan using language that is culturally sensitive and at an appropriate reading level to be understood by all participants.

- Uses standardized terminology to document the plan.

Additional Measurement Criteria for the Advanced Practice Public Health Nurse:

The advanced practice public health nurse:

- Applies assessment, implementation, and evaluation strategies in the plan to reflect current evidence, including data, research, literature, and expert nursing and public health knowledge.

The content in this appendix is not current and is of historical significance only.

- Designs appropriate strategies and alternatives with community and professional partners to meet the complex needs of at-risk populations.

- Incorporates population values and beliefs with community and professional partners in the planning process.

- Leads other public health nurses and the multi-sector team in the use of principles of planning for population-focused programs and services.

- Contributes to the development and continuous improvement of organizational systems that support the planning process.

- Participates in the integration of human, fiscal, material, scientific, and population resources to enhance and complete the planning process for programs or services.

- Assures that the current standards, statutes, regulations, and policies are considered in the planning process.

The content in this appendix is not current and is of historical significance only.

STANDARD 5. IMPLEMENTATION
The public health nurse implements the identified plan by partnering with others.

Measurement Criteria:

The public health nurse:

- Implements the identified plan in a safe and timely manner in collaboration with the multi-sector team.

- Applies evidence-based strategies and activities, including opportunities for coalition building and advocacy, in a plan that is specific to the population assets, needs, and concerns.

- Incorporates systems and population resources in implementing the plan.

- Monitors implementation of the plan, including processes and resource utilization.

- Documents implementation of the plan, including modifications.

Additional Measurement Criteria for the Advanced Practice Public Health Nurse:

The advanced practice public health nurse:

- Interprets surveillance data related to the plan and population health status.

- Incorporates new knowledge and strategies into action plans to enhance implementation.

- Modifies the plan based on new knowledge, appropriate health behavior change theory, population response, or other relevant factors to achieve expected outcomes.

- Advocates for bringing needed resources to the community and for the population to implement the plan.

- Fosters new collaborative relationships with nursing colleagues, other professionals, community or population representatives, and other stakeholders to implement the plan through strategies such as coalition building.

- Promotes organizations, community coalitions, and systems that support the plan.

The content in this appendix is not current and is of historical significance only.

STANDARD 5A. COORDINATION

The public health nurse coordinates programs, services, and other activities to implement the identified plan.

Measurement Criteria:

The public health nurse:

- Promotes policies, programs, and services for the attainment of expected outcomes.

- Conducts surveillance, case finding, and reporting functions with health professionals and other stakeholders.

- Connects populations with needed services.

- Documents the coordination and required reporting.

Additional Measurement Criteria for the Advanced Practice Public Health Nurse:

The advanced practice public health nurse:

- Provides leadership for delivery of integrated programs, services, and public policy implementation.

- Synthesizes data and information to initiate system, community, and environmental resource allocation that support the delivery of programs and services.

The content in this appendix is not current and is of historical significance only.

STANDARD 5B. HEALTH EDUCATION AND HEALTH PROMOTION

The public health nurse employs multiple strategies to promote health, prevent disease, and ensure a safe environment for populations.

Measurement Criteria:

The public health nurse:

- Includes appropriate health education in the implementation of programs and services for populations.

- Selects teaching and learning methods appropriate to the health literacy of the population and their identified objectives.

- Presents culturally and age-appropriate health promotion, disease prevention, and environmental safety information and educational materials to the population.

- Collects feedback from participants to determine program and service effectiveness and recommended changes.

Additional Measurement Criteria for the Advanced Practice Public Health Nurse:

The advanced practice public health nurse:

- Provides leadership to nursing and other health professionals in planning evidence-based educational programs and services based on assessments.

- Designs health information and programs based on health behavior, learning theories and principles, and research evidence.

- Modifies existing programs based on feedback from participants, providers, health professionals, and other stakeholders.

- Develops health information resources that are culturally and age-appropriate to the population.

The content in this appendix is not current and is of historical significance only.

Standard 5c. Consultation

The public health nurse provides consultation to various community groups and officials to facilitate the implementation of programs and services.

Measurement Criteria:

The public health nurse:

- Confers with community organizations and groups to facilitate participation in programs and services.

- Provides testimony and professional opinion on programs and service delivery to at-risk populations.

- Communicates effectively using a variety of media with constituent groups during consultation.

- Documents the scope and effectiveness of consultation activities provided to community populations.

Additional Measurement Criteria for the Advanced Practice Public Health Nurse:

The advanced practice public health nurse:

- Synthesizes data from federal, state, local, and other sources with theoretical frameworks and evidence, to provide expert consultation on program and service implementation.

- Provides expert testimony at the federal, state, and local levels on program and service delivery to at-risk populations.

- Communicates information during consultation toward a positive influence on the provision of programs and services to populations.

- Generates proposals and reports in support of needed programs and services.

The content in this appendix is not current and is of historical significance only.

STANDARD 5D. REGULATORY ACTIVITIES
The public health nurse identifies, interprets, and implements public health laws, regulations, and policies.

Measurement Criteria:

The public health nurse:

- Educates affected populations on relevant laws, regulations, and policies.

- Participates in the application of public health laws, regulations, and policies, including monitoring and inspecting regulated entities.

- Collects specific information about situations that are reported to public health officials.

- Assists in addressing non-compliance with laws, regulations, and policies.

Additional Measurement Criteria for the Advanced Practice Public Health Nurse:

The advanced practice public health nurse:

- Collaborates in the revision or development of public health laws, regulations, and policies.

- Designs, with other public health professionals, reporting and compliance systems related to laws, regulations, and policies.

- Monitors reporting and compliance systems for quality and appropriate use of resources.

- Analyzes data from reporting and compliance systems.

- Develops reports for public health officials and other decision-makers as required by laws, regulations, and policies.

- Participates in coordinating emergency preparedness and response efforts, including receipt and use of the Strategic National Stockpile.

The content in this appendix is not current and is of historical significance only.

STANDARD 6. EVALUATION
The public health nurse evaluates the health status of the population.

Measurement Criteria:

The public health nurse:

- Participates in a systematic, ongoing, and criterion-based evaluation of service outcomes with the population and other stakeholders.

- Collects data systematically, applying epidemiological and scientific methods to determine the effectiveness of public health nursing interventions on policies, programs, and services.

- Participates in process and outcome evaluation by monitoring activities in programs or services.

- Applies ongoing assessment data to revise plans, interventions, and activities, as appropriate.

- Documents the results of the evaluation including changes or recommendations to enhance effectiveness of interventions.

- Disseminates the process and outcome evaluation results to the population and other stakeholders in accordance with state and federal laws and regulations, as appropriate.

Additional Measurement Criteria for the Advanced Practice Public Health Nurse:

The advanced practice public health nurse:

- Designs an evaluation plan with other public health experts, and with representatives from the population and from stakeholders.

- Modifies the evaluation plan for policies, programs, or services, as appropriate.

- Evaluates the effectiveness of the plan in relationship to expected and unexpected outcomes.

- Synthesizes the results of the evaluation analyses to determine the effect of the plan on populations, organizations, and other stakeholder groups.

- Applies the results of the evaluation analyses to recommend or make process or outcomes changes in policies, programs, or services, as appropriate.

The content in this appendix is not current and is of historical significance only.

STANDARDS OF PROFESSIONAL PERFORMANCE

STANDARD 7. QUALITY OF PRACTICE
The public health nurse systematically enhances the quality and effectiveness of nursing practice.

Measurement Criteria:

The public health nurse:

- Demonstrates quality through the application of the nursing process in a responsible, accountable, and ethical manner.

- Implements new knowledge and performance improvement activities to initiate changes in public health nursing practice and in the delivery of care to populations.

- Incorporates creativity and innovation in activities to improve the quality of nursing practice.

- Participates in the development, implementation, and evaluation of procedures and guidelines to improve the quality of practice.

- Participates in the scope of the performance improvement activities as appropriate to the nurse's position, education, and practice environment. Such activities may include:

  - Identifying aspects of practice important for quality monitoring.

  - Employing evidence-based indicators to monitor the quality and effectiveness of nursing practice.

  - Collecting data to monitor public health nursing practice, including availability, accessibility, acceptability, quality, and effectiveness of policies, programs, and services.

  - Monitoring indicators of quality and effectiveness of policies, programs, and services.

  - Analyzing the data to identify opportunities for improving nursing practice.

  - Formulating recommendations to improve nursing practice or outcomes.

Continued ▶

The content in this appendix is not current and is of historical significance only.

- Implementing activities to enhance the quality of nursing practice.

- Participating with the population and other professionals, organizations, and stakeholders in the evaluation of policies, programs, and services.

- Assessing professional performance factors related to population safety, accessibility to services, program effectiveness, and cost–benefit options.

- Analyzing organization and program processes and systems to remove or decrease barriers and to enhance assets.

- Documents the delivery of programs and services in ways that reflect the quality measures.

- Obtains and maintains professional certification, if available, in the area of expertise.

Additional Measurement Criteria for the Advanced Practice Public Health Nurse:

The advanced practice public health nurse:

- Designs performance improvement initiatives related to policies, programs, and services based on existing evidence.

- Implements initiatives to evaluate the need for change.

- Evaluates the practice environment and quality of nursing care rendered in relation to existing evidence-based information.

- Identifies opportunities for the generation and use of research to enhance the evidence base for public health nursing practice.

The content in this appendix is not current and is of historical significance only.

STANDARD 8. EDUCATION
The public health nurse attains knowledge and competency that reflects current nursing and public health practice.

Measurement Criteria:

The public health nurse:

- Participates in ongoing educational activities to maintain and enhance the knowledge and skills necessary to promote the health of the population.

- Seeks experiences to develop and maintain competence in the skills needed to implement policies, programs, and services for populations.

- Identifies learning needs based on nursing and public health knowledge, the various roles the nurse may assume, and the changing needs of the population.

- Identifies changes in the statutory requirements for the practice of nursing and public health.

- Maintains professional records that provide evidence of competency and lifelong learning.

- Seeks experiences and formal and independent learning activities to maintain and develop clinical and professional skills and knowledge.

Additional Measurement Criteria for the Advanced Practice Public Health Nurse:

The advanced practice public health nurse:

- Uses current research findings and other evidence to expand nursing and public health knowledge, enhance role performance, and increase knowledge of professional issues.

The content in this appendix is not current and is of historical significance only.

STANDARD 9. PROFESSIONAL PRACTICE EVALUATION

The public health nurse evaluates one's own nursing practice in relation to professional practice standards and guidelines, relevant statutes, rules, and regulations.

Measurement Criteria:

The public health nurse:

- Implements age-appropriate population-focused policies, programs, and services in a culturally and ethnically sensitive manner.

- Engages in self-evaluation of practice on a regular basis, identifying areas of strength as well as areas in which professional development would be beneficial.

- Seeks feedback regarding one's own practice from community and professional partners and other peers.

- Implements plans for accomplishing goals in one's own work plan.

- Integrates the knowledge of current practice standards, guidelines, statutes, rules, and regulations into one's own work plans.

- Provides rationale for professional practice beliefs, decisions, and actions as part of the evaluation process.

- Applies knowledge of current practice standards, guidelines, statutes, certification, and regulation in self-evaluation and peer review.

Additional Measurement Criteria for the Advanced Practice Public Health Nurse:

The advanced practice public health nurse:

- Engages in a formal systematic process seeking feedback regarding one's own practice from peers, professional colleagues, community and professional organizations, and stakeholders.

- Analyzes practice in relation to advanced certification requirements as appropriate.

The content in this appendix is not current and is of historical significance only.

STANDARD 10. COLLEGIALITY AND PROFESSIONAL RELATIONSHIPS

The public health nurse establishes collegial partnerships while interacting with representatives of the population, organizations, and health and human services professionals, and contributes to the professional development of peers, students, colleagues, and others.

Measurement Criteria:

The public health nurse:

- Shares knowledge and skills with peers, students, colleagues, and others.

- Interacts with peers, students, colleagues, and others to enhance professional nursing or public health practice and role performance of self and others.

- Mentors other public health nurses, colleagues, students, and others as appropriate.

- Maintains compassionate and caring relationships with professional colleagues and other stakeholders involved in population health.

- Contributes to an environment that fosters ongoing educational experiences for colleagues, healthcare professionals, and the population.

- Contributes to a supportive, healthy, and safe work environment.

Additional Measurement Criteria for the Advanced Practice Public Health Nurse:

The advanced practice public health nurse:

- Models expert practice to multi-sector team members and the population.

- Designs mentoring policies and programs for public health nurses and other colleagues.

- Participates in activities that contribute to the development of the advanced practice nursing role in public health.

The content in this appendix is not current and is of historical significance only.

STANDARD 11. COLLABORATION

The public health nurse collaborates with representatives of the population, organizations, and health and human service professionals in providing for and promoting the health of the population.

Measurement Criteria:

The public health nurse:

- Communicates with various constituencies in the community to gather information and develop partnerships and coalitions to address population-focused health concerns.

- Partners with individuals, groups, and community-based organizations in the assessment, planning, implementing, and evaluation of population-focused policies, programs, and services.

- Articulates nursing and public health knowledge and skills to the interdisciplinary team, administrators, policy-makers, and other multi-sector partners.

- Partners with other disciplines in teaching, program development and implementation, evaluation, research, and public policy advocacy.

- Contributes to the multi-sector team in implementing public health regulatory requirements such as case identification, program management, and mandatory reporting.

- Partners with key individuals, groups, coalitions, and organizations to effect change in public health policies, programs, and services to generate positive outcomes.

- Documents collaborative interactions and processes related to policies, programs, and services.

Additional Measurement Criteria for the Advanced Practice Public Health Nurse:

The advanced practice public health nurse:

- Develops alliances and coalitions with community organizations to address public health policies, programs, and services.

- Initiates collaborative efforts across constituencies in the population.

The content in this appendix is not current and is of historical significance only.

- Designs educational, administrative, research, and public policy programs to promote the health of the population.

- Develops systems for documentation and accountability in nursing and public health nursing practice, including compliance with regulatory requirements.

The content in this appendix is not current and is of historical significance only.

STANDARD 12. ETHICS
The public health nurse integrates ethical provisions in all areas of practice.

Measurement Criteria:

The public health nurse:

- Applies *Code of Ethics for Nurses with Interpretive Statements* (ANA, 2001) and *Principles of the Ethical Practice of Public Health* (Public Health Leadership Society, 2002) to guide public health nursing practice.

- Delivers programs and services in a manner that preserves, protects, and promotes the autonomy, dignity, and rights of the population or community as well as individuals.

- Applies ethical standards in advocating for health and social policy.

- Maintains individual confidentiality within legal and regulatory parameters.

- Assists populations, communities, and individuals in developing skills for self-advocacy.

- Maintains professional relationships and boundaries with individuals and groups within the population while delivering public health services and programs.

- Demonstrates a commitment to fostering an environment and conditions in which healthy lifestyles may be practiced by self, colleagues, and identified populations.

- Contributes to resolving social and environmental issues and barriers to healthy living conditions.

- Contributes to resolving ethical issues involving colleagues, community groups, systems, and other stakeholders.

- Reports activities that are illegal, inconsistent with accepted standards of practice, or reflective of impaired practice.

The content in this appendix is not current and is of historical significance only.

Additional Measurement Criteria for the Advanced Practice Public Health Nurse:

The advanced practice public health nurse:

- Informs populations and communities of the risks, benefits, and outcomes of policies, programs, and services.

- Informs administrators or others of the risks, benefits, and outcomes of policies, programs, and services, and related decisions that affect the delivery of health-related services.

- Partners with multi-sector teams to address ethical risks, benefits, and outcomes of policies, programs, and services.

- Promotes solutions to social and environmental issues and barriers to healthy living conditions.

The content in this appendix is not current and is of historical significance only.

STANDARD 13. RESEARCH
The public health nurse integrates research findings into practice.

Measurement Criteria:

The public health nurse:

- Utilizes the best available evidence, including research findings, to guide practice, policy, and service delivery decisions.

- Actively participates in research activities at various levels appropriate to one's own level of education and position. Such activities may include:

  - Identifying community and professional opportunities suitable for nursing and public health research.

  - Participating in data collection.

  - Participating in agency-, organization-, or population-focused research committees or programs.

  - Sharing research activities and findings with peers and others.

  - Implementing research protocols.

  - Critically analyzing and interpreting research for application to population-focused practice.

  - Applying nursing and public health research findings in the development of policies, programs, and services for populations.

  - Incorporating research as a basis for learning.

- Actively involves communities, populations, organizations, and other stakeholder groups in a participatory research process.

Additional Measurement Criteria for the Advanced Practice Public Health Nurse:

The advanced practice public health nurse:

- Contributes to nursing knowledge by conducting or synthesizing research that discovers, examines, and evaluates knowledge, theories, models, criteria, and creative approaches to improve healthcare practice and outcomes.

- Formally disseminates research findings through consultation, presentations, publications, and the use of other media.

The content in this appendix is not current and is of historical significance only.

STANDARD 14. RESOURCE UTILIZATION
The public health nurse considers factors related to safety, effectiveness, cost, and impact on practice and on the population in the planning and delivery of nursing and public health programs, policies, and services.

Measurement Criteria:

The public health nurse:

- Evaluates factors such as safety, effectiveness, availability, cost and benefits, efficiencies, and impact on practice and on the population, when choosing practice options that would result in the same expected outcome.

- Assists representatives of specific populations and other stakeholders in identifying and securing appropriate and available services to address health-related needs.

- Assigns or delegates tasks taking into consideration the concerns of the population, potential for harm, complexity of the task, and predictability of the outcomes.

- Helps the population to become informed about the options, costs, risks, and benefits of policies, programs, and services.

Additional Measurement Criteria for the Advanced Practice Public Health Nurse:

The advanced practice public health nurse:

- Utilizes organizational and community resources to formulate multi-sector plans for policies, programs, and services.

- Develops innovative approaches to community and public health concerns that include effective resource utilization and improvement of quality.

- Develops evaluation strategies to demonstrate cost effectiveness and efficiency factors associated with nursing and public health practice and outcomes.

The content in this appendix is not current and is of historical significance only.

STANDARD 15. LEADERSHIP
The public health nurse provides leadership in nursing and public health.

Measurement Criteria:

The public health nurse:

- Engages in multi-sector team development and coalition building, including other professionals, the population, and stakeholders.

- Promotes healthy community and work environments at local, regional, national, and international levels.

- Articulates the mission, goals, action plan, and outcome measures of nursing and public health programs and services to other professionals and the population.

- Advocates for opportunities for continuous, lifelong learning for self and others.

- Teaches peers, stakeholders, and others in the population to succeed through mentoring and other strategies.

- Exhibits creativity and flexibility through times of change.

- Fosters a culture where systems are monitored and evaluated to improve the quality of policies, programs, and services for populations.

- Coordinates programs and services across various community settings and among the multi-sector team.

- Serves in leadership roles in the work setting, in the community, and with the population.

- Promotes advancement of public health and nursing through participation in professional organizations.

- Functions as a public health team leader in emergency preparedness and response situations, delegating tasks as delineated in standardized protocols.

The content in this appendix is not current and is of historical significance only.

Additional Measurement Criteria for the Advanced Practice Public Health Nurse:

The advanced practice public health nurse:

- Advocates with decision-makers to influence public health policies, programs, and services to promote healthy populations.

- Provides direction to enhance the effectiveness of policies, programs, and services provided by the multi-sector team.

- Initiates and revises protocols or guidelines to reflect evidence-based practice, to reflect accepted changes in program and service delivery, or to address emerging problems in the population.

- Promotes communication of information and advancement of nursing and public health through writing, publishing, and presentations for professional or lay audiences.

- Demonstrates innovative approaches to public health and nursing practice to improve health outcomes for populations.

- Organizes formal plans in response to public health emergencies for populations.

The content in this appendix is not current and is of historical significance only.

STANDARD 16. ADVOCACY

The public health nurse advocates to protect the health, safety, and rights of the population.

Measurement Criteria:

The public health nurse:

- Incorporates the identified needs of the population in policy development and program or service planning.

- Integrates advocacy into the implementation of policies, programs, and services for the population.

- Evaluates the effectiveness of advocating for the population when assessing the expected outcomes.

- Includes confidentiality, ethical, legal, privacy, and professional guidelines in policy development and other issues.

- Demonstrates skill in advocating before providers and stakeholders on behalf of the population.

- Strives to resolve conflicting expectations from populations, providers, and other stakeholders to ensure the safety and to guard the best interest of the population and to preserve the professional integrity of the nurse.

Additional Measurement Criteria for the Advanced Practice Public Health Nurse:

The advanced practice public health nurse:

- Demonstrates skill in advocating before public representatives and decision-makers on behalf of the populations, programs, and services.

- Designs materials for the advocacy process that are based on the needs of the populations, programs, and services.

- Exhibits fiscal responsibility and integrity in the policy development process.

- Serves as an expert for peers, populations, providers, and other stakeholders in promoting and implementing public health policies.

The content in this appendix is not current and is of historical significance only.

GLOSSARY

Advocacy. The act of pleading or arguing in favor of a cause, idea, or policy on someone else's behalf, with the object of developing the community, system, individual, or family's capacity to plead their own cause or act on their own behalf.

Assessment. The regular and systematic collection, analysis, and dissemination of information on the health of the community or population, including statistics on health status, community health needs, and epidemiological and other studies of health problems.

Assurance. Assuring that services necessary to achieve agreed-upon goals are provided by encouraging actions by other entities (private or public), by requiring such action through regulation, or by providing services directly.

Coalition building. The process by which parties (individuals, organizations, or groups) come together to form a temporary alliance or union to work together for a common purpose and to enhance each other's capacity for mutual benefit and common purpose.

Collaboration. Work with another person or group to achieve some end.

Community. A set of persons in interaction, being and experiencing together, who may or may not share a sense of place or belonging, and who act intentionally for a common purpose. A community is different from the group of people who constitute it and can interact with other entities as a unit.

Community-based organizations. Private nonprofit organizations or other types of groups that work within a community for the improvement of some aspect of that community.

Cultural competence. A set of congruent behaviors, attitudes, and policies that come together in a system or agency or among professionals and enable the system, agency, or professionals to work effectively in cross-cultural settings.

Cultural diversity. The coexistence of different ethnic, gender, racial, and socioeconomic groups.

The content in this appendix is not current and is of historical significance only.

Determinants of health. Social, economic, and healthcare factors that affect health and well-being independently or in conjunction with each other at the population or community level. Comprehensive factors involve relevant social, economic, environmental, behavioral, political, health, and healthcare indicators that describe the essential features of a social structure and system and the processes through which change occurs.

Ecological model. A model of health that emphasizes the linkages and relationships among multiple factors (or determinants) affecting health.

Environmental health. Those aspects of human health, including quality of life, that are determined by physical, chemical, biological, social, and psychological processes in the environment. It also refers to the theory and practice of assessing, correcting, controlling, or preventing those factors in the environment that can adversely affect the health of the present and future generations.

Epidemiology. The study of the distribution of determinants and antecedents of health and disease in human populations. The ultimate goal is to identify the underlying causes of a disease and then to apply those findings to disease prevention and health promotion.

Evidence. Verifiable knowledge on which belief is based.

Evidence-based practice. An approach to public healthcare practice in which the public health nurse is aware of the evidence in support of one's clinical practice, and the strength of that evidence.

Health status (of a population). The level of illness or wellness of a population at a designated time.

Interdisciplinary team. A group of individuals who rely on each other's overlapping skills and discipline-based knowledge to achieve synergistic effects where outcomes are enhanced and more comprehensive than the simple aggregation of individual members' efforts.

Multi-sector team. A partnership of community organizations and groups representing a variety of viewpoints and perspectives which impact public health issues.

Outcomes. Long-term objectives that define optimal, measurable future levels of health status, maximum acceptable levels of disease, injury, or dysfunction, or prevalence of risk factors.

The content in this appendix is not current and is of historical significance only.

Partnership. A relationship in which two or more people or groups operate together to achieve a common goal.

Performance improvement. A process that considers the organizational context, describes desired performance, identifies gaps between desired and actual performance, identifies root causes, selects interventions to close the gaps, and measures changes in performance with the goal of achieving desired results or outcomes.

Policy development. Applying comprehensive public health scientific knowledge for decision-making. Policy development includes a systematic course of action to establish priorities, determine effective strategies and interventions, and use community resources, including regulation and law, to achieve the community's goals.

Population. Those living in a specific geographic area (e.g., a neighborhood, community, city, or county) or those in a particular group (e.g., racial, ethnic, age) who experience a disproportionate burden of poor health outcomes.

Population-focused. An approach to health care that operates at the population level of the ecological model.

Priorities. A ranking or ordering of diagnoses, strategies, or activities that identifies those that are most important or that should be addressed first.

Social justice. The principle that all persons are entitled to have their basic human needs met, regardless of differences in economic status, class, gender, race, ethnicity, citizenship, religion, age, sexual orientation, disability, or health. This includes the eradication of poverty and illiteracy, the establishment of sound environmental policy, and equality of opportunity for healthy personal and social development.

Stakeholder. A person or organization that has a legitimate interest in what a public health entity does.

Standard. An authoritative statement, defined and promoted by the profession, by which the quality of practice, service, or education can be evaluated.

Strategic national stockpile. Large quantities of medicines, antidotes, and medical supples needed to respond to a wide range of circumstances where supplies of critical medical items in any jurisdiction would

The content in this appendix is not current and is of historical significance only.

be rapidly depleted; the stockpile is managed by the Centers for Disease Control and Prevention (CDC).

Surveillance. The systematic collection, analysis, interpretation, and dissemination of data to assist in the planning, implementation, and evaluation of public health interventions and programs.

The content in this appendix is not current and is of historical significance only.

REFERENCES

American Nurses Association (ANA). (1973). *Standards of nursing practice.* Washington, DC: American Nurses Publishing. (Also available as appendix in ANA 2004a.)

American Nurses Association (ANA). (1986). *Standards of community nursing practice.* Washington, DC: American Nurses Publishing.

American Nurses Association (ANA). (1999). *Scope and standards of public health nursing.* Washington, DC: American Nurses Publishing.

American Nurses Association (ANA). (2001). *Code of ethics for nurses with interpretive statements.* Washington, DC: American Nurses Publishing.

American Nurses Association (ANA). (2003). *Nursing's social policy statement, 2nd edition.* Washington, DC: Nursesbooks.org.

American Nurses Association (ANA). (2004a). *Nursing: Scope and standards of practice.* Silver Spring, MD: Nursesbooks.org.

American Nurses Association (ANA). (2004b). *Scope and standards for nurse administrators, 2nd edition.* Silver Spring, MD: Nursesbooks.org.

American Public Health Association (APHA). Public Health Nursing Section (PHNS). (1996). The definition and role of public health nursing. Retrieved August 23, 2005, from http://www.csuchico.edu/~horst/about/definition.html.

American Public Health Association (APHA). Public Health Nursing Section (PHNS). (2006). Environmental health principles and recommendations for public health nursing. Washington, DC: APHA

Association of Community Health Nursing Educators (ACHNE). (2000). *Essentials of baccalaureate nursing education for entry level community health nursing practice.* Latham, NY: ACHNE.

The content in this appendix is not current and is of historical significance only.

Association of Community Health Nursing Educators (ACHNE). (2003). *Essentials of master's level nursing education for advanced community/ public health nursing practice.* Latham, NY: ACHNE.

Centers for Disease Control and Prevention (CDC). (2001). *National public health performance standards.* Retrieved August 23, 2005, from http://www.cdc.gov/od/ocphp/nphpsp/TheInstruments.htm.

Council on Linkages Between Academia and Public Health Practice. (2001). *Core competencies for public health professionals.* Retrieved August 23, 2005, from http://www.phf.org/competencies.htm.

Department of Health and Human Services (HHS). (2000). *Healthy people 2010, 2nd edition.* Washington, DC: U.S. Government Printing Office.

Institute of Medicine (IOM). (1988). *The future of public health.* Washington, DC: National Academies Press.

Institute of Medicine (IOM). (1995). *Nursing, health, and the environment.* Washington, DC: National Academies Press.

Institute of Medicine (IOM). (2003a). *The future of the public's health in the twenty-first century.* Washington, DC: National Academies Press.

Institute of Medicine (IOM). (2003b). *Who will keep the public healthy?* Washington, DC: National Academies Press.

Public Health Leadership Society. (2002). *Principles of the ethical practice of public health, version 2.2.* Retrieved August 23, 2005, from http://www.phls.org.

Quad Council of Public Health Nursing Organizations. (2004). Public health nursing competencies. *Public Health Nursing, 21*(5), 443–452.

Quad Council of Public Health Nursing Organizations & American Nurses Association. (1999). *Scope and standards of public health nursing practice.* Washington, DC: American Nurses Publishing.

The content in this appendix is not current and is of historical significance only.

Tickner, J. (2002). Precaution and preventive public health policy. *Policy Health Reports, 117*, 493–497.

Tickner, J., & Raffensberger, C. (1998). *The precautionary principle in action: A handbook, 1st edition*. Retrieved August 16, 2006, from http://www.sehn.org/rtfdocs/handbook-rtf.rtf.

APPENDIX A
COMPARISON OF MULTIPLE DETERMINANTS OF POPULATION HEALTH USING AN ECOLOGICAL FRAMEWORK AND SELECTED PUBLIC HEALTH NURSING INTERVENTION MODELS

An ecological framework for guiding public health nursing interventions considers multiple determinants of population health (individual behavior; social, family, and community networks of support; living and working conditions; and policies) in conjunction with the levels of potential influence (macro-upstream, midlevel, micro-downstream, and proximate) on those determinants.

References

ASTDN Model
Association of State and Territorial Directors of Nursing (ASTDN) and American Nurses Association (ANA). (2000). *Public health nursing: A partner for healthy populations*. Washington, DC: American Nurses Publishing.

EPI Model
Koepsell, T. D., & N. S. Weiss. (2003). *Diseases and populations in epidemiologic methods*, pp. 17–36. New York: Oxford University Press.

Laffrey and Kulbok Model
Laffrey, S. C., & P. A. Kulbok. (1999). An integrative model for holistic community health nursing. *Journal of Holistic Nursing 17*(1): 88–103.

MN Model
Keller, L. O., S. Strohschein, B. Lia-Hoagberg, & M. A. Schaffer. (2004). Population-based public health interventions: Practice-based and evidence supported. *Public Health Nursing 21*(5): 453–468 (September).

Salmon Model
Salmon, M. E. (1993). Public health nursing: The opportunity of a lifetime. *American Journal of Public Health 83*(1): 674–675.

The content in this appendix is not current and is of historical significance only.

Determinant Category / Intervention Model	Individual	Social, Family, and Community	Living and Working Conditions	Broad Social, Economic, Cultural, Health, Environmental Conditions and Policies
Anderson/McFarlane Model Community as Partner	Communities are composed of individuals, who are considered as equal partners with the nurse in this model. The community's people are at the core of the model.	The model begins with a community assessment wheel, considering the core (demography, values, beliefs, and history) and eight subsystem components, of which health and social services is one. Communities have a normal line of defense (health); a flexible line of defense (buffer zone); and a line of resistance. The degree of reaction to stressors becomes part of the nursing diagnosis.	Components of the subsystems of a community include the physical environment, safety and transportation, communication, economics, and recreation. Living and working conditions are considered across more than one of these subsystems as defined in this model.	The healthy community functions in equilibrium within its normal line of defense. Disequilibrium occurs when internal or external stressors (temporary or permanent) are introduced. The community responds to stressors based on its previous patterns of coping and problem-solving capabilities, in the context of this model.
ASTDN Model (Association of State and Territorial Directors of Nursing)	Care of the individual provides a foundation for population health practice through the application of knowledge to the aggregate.	Families and communities are served through fluid activity between nursing practice (critical thinking, the nursing process, a holistic approach) and the Core Public Health Functions and Essential Services.	The nurse acts on conditions in the environment through critical thinking and the nursing process by performing the duties of the Essential Public Health Services.	The practice of nursing and the Core Public Health Functions provide a framework for organizing, delivering, and evaluating interventions aimed at improving health with the Essential Public Health Services further delineating the functions.
EPI Model	**Multifactorial human–environment interaction:** Individual effects are influenced by varying emphasis of individual (genetics, biology) and environmental (physical, social, biological) factors.	Existing biological and genetic factors in a family or community interact with social, physical, and biological factors in the environment to determine health outcomes.	**Multiple ecological interactions:** The health impact of biological, social, and physical factors in the environment varies by the public health problem or disease under consideration.	**Multiple ecological interactions:** Social, physical, and biological manipulation of the environment affect health. Measures for controlling disease or improving health can be evaluated in terms of the total effect on the ecosystem and human health.

The content in this appendix is not current and is of historical significance only.

Laffrey & Kulbok (1999), *Integrative Model For Community Health Promotion*	**Multidimensional Client Systems:** Individual most delimited level **Focus of Care (across all client systems):** Health Promotion, Illness Prevention, and Illness Care. The goal of C/PHN is a healthy community, achieved through health promotion interventions. No matter where C/PHN care begins, it ultimately leads to health promotion of the community.	**Client System:** Family, aggregate, and community	Each successive client system or level provides the environment for the preceding level. Family, aggregate, and community compose the environment for the individual level; aggregate and community make up the environment for the family, and the community is the environment for the aggregate. Different kinds of interventions are appropriate at each level of client within the system.	**Client System:** Increasingly complex from delimited individual system to complex community and society C/PHN is holistic in nature and is population-focused in that it addresses multiple levels of client and multiple levels of care within the total system.
MN Model *PHN Interventions*	Three levels of practice are defined in the population-based model. Interventions at the individual level focus on changing attitudes, knowledge, beliefs, practices, and behaviors. These interventions contribute to the overall goal of improving population health. Interventions of particular relevance to this level of practice include referral, case management, health teaching, counseling, and consultation.		Population-based community practice changes community norms, community attitudes, community awareness, practices, and behaviors. Interventions that may have particular relevance at this level include collaboration, coalition building, and community organizing. In addition, surveillance and screening are particularly critical to maintaining health in a community.	Population systems-focused practice changes organizations, policies, laws, and power structure. The focus of practice is on systems that affect health. Interventions that may be particularly relevant to this practice include advocacy, social marketing, and policy development, as well as collaboration and organizing.
Salmon Model	The individual is the point at which the continuum of intervention by the public health nurse begins. There are human and biological determinants of health which affect the individual's contribution to the health status continuum. The public health nurse must understand and consider these as one element of the construct for practice.	Social determinants of health are a category of focus in this model. Valuing of the public good lies at the ethical core of this model. The public health nurse considers interventions that affect social and political processes, with prevention being the primary focus.	Environmental determinants of health are one of the four categories of factors affecting the health of the public which the public health nurse considers in carrying out the nursing process. Environmental factors, like the other three determinants, are considered at individual, group, community, family, and population levels.	This model describes medical, technological, and organizational determinants of health as the fourth category. This category considers the organization of the total healthcare system. Public health nursing interventions are targeted and intentional, based on consideration of all four aspects of the construct.

Index

Note: Entries with [2007] indicate an entry from *Public Health Nursing: Scope and Standards of Practice* (2007), reproduced in Appendix B. That information is not current but included for historical value only. Page numbers followed by "f" indicate reference to a figure.

A